THRIVING *WITH* ILLNESS

DENNIS O'BRIEN

Thriving With Illness
Dennis O'Brien

First published in Australia by Dennis O'Brien 2023
Copyright © O'Brien 2023
All Rights Reserved

A catalogue record for this
book is available from the
National Library of Australia

ISBN: 978-0-6458804-0-3 (pbk)
ISBN: 978-0-6458804-1-0 (ebk)

Typesetting and design by Publicious Book Publishing
Published in collaboration with Publicious Book
Publishing. www.publicious.com.au

No part of this book may be reproduced in any form,
by photocopying or by any electronic or mechanical
means, including information storage or retrieval
systems, without permission in writing from both the
copyright owner and the publisher of this book.

Dedication

I dedicate this book to my wife Deborah who has stood by me in all of my career endeavours and also has been my carer during my many spells in hospital and in recuperating afterwards. She has had to deal with me being in a wheelchair on several occasions, a period of insanity and various spell of serious illness.

Deborah is a born organiser and makes sure our lives are fully occupied with travel and, when at home frequent meals with friends. Her skills in this area also extend to the community where she is President of the local View Club.

Table of Contents

Chapter 1. In Hospital Again 1

Chapter 2.
    Extract from Australian Pituitary
    Foundation Web Site. 11
    INCIDENCE 11
    PREVALENCE 11
    ABOUT CUSHING'S DISEASE 11
    PRESENTING SIGNS AND SYMPTOMS 12
    Cushing's disease can be difficult to diagnose as
    some of the symptoms are very common in the
    general population and occur with other medical
    conditions. Further, symptoms and signs can develop
    slowly over long periods of time, making Cushing's
    disease even harder to recognise. 12
    INVESTIGATIONS 13
    TREATMENT 14
    AFTER SURGERY 16
    LONG-TERM OUTCOMES 17
    COMMON QUESTIONS 18

Chapter 3.
    Cushing's Experiences of the Author 20
    My case 20
    Hardening of Arteries 21
    Time to Diagnose and Morbidity 22
    A Not So Rare Disease 22

Chapter 4. My Father 23

Chapter 5. My Mother 28

Chapter 6. My upbringing. 30

Chapter 7. Cadetship 1971 to 1977 45

Chapter 8. NDY Queensland 1977 to 1987 51

Chapter 9. NDY New Zealand 1997 to 1990 60

Chapter 10. NDY Sydney 1990 to 2007. 66

Chapter 11. Various Locations 2007 to 2009. 104

Chapter 12. Gold Coast 2009 to 2013. 133

Chapter 13. Gold Coast 2013 to 2023. 151

Chapter 14.
- Rantings of an Old Man. 163
- How I Have Changed. 163
- Treatment of disabled people. 165
- People who inspire. 166
- Our Health System 168
- Rare Diseases. 168

Chapter 15. The Future. 170

Acknowledgements 175

Chapter 1. In Hospital Again

In November 2022, I found myself back in Pindara Hospital on the Gold Coast. I think I should qualify for Frequent Flyer points given my regular stays, but they do look after me very well. This is one of many spells in various hospitals between 2009 and now. Another battle in my ongoing war with the Devil.

Now before you call me crazy, let me explain how this came about. I have undergone a lot of management and personal training and one of the techniques I learned is to find the inspiration to carry out a task which may otherwise be boring or unpleasant. The reason does not have to be true or logical, but it must be one that inspires you.

After many years of illness, I was diagnosed with Cushing's Disease in 2013. I was by this time in very poor shape physically and mentally. There was extensive testing required to establish what was happening and during this time I suffered from psychosis which is not uncommon with Cushing's.

I one of my training courses, I had learned a technique to adopt when I was confronted with a task or a situation which might be considered boring or unpleasant. The trick is to find a reason or purpose for the situation which is inspiring.

Chapter 1 – In Hospital Again

In my confused state, I decided that the best reason to fight the disease was to visualise that the Devil was responsible and there was no way I would let the bastard win. I am not a religious person, but it seemed at the time this would be the best rallying call on which I would face the challenges ahead of me. I honestly don't know that I would have adopted this "reason" if I had been sane at the time. However, it did work for me, and I keep it in mind each time I face one of the many challenges the disease seems to impose on sufferers.

My wife Deborah and I recently returned from a holiday which included catching the Ghan from Darwin to Adelaide. I had a sore toe prior to leaving but was unable to get medical attention so put up with it for the trip.

I visited my GP on my return, and she diagnosed an ulcer which Cushing's predisposes me to. I have suffered many infections of this type. More seriously, it was discovered that the 3 major arteries in the leg were blocked which would be a key reason the ulcer occurred. It also prevented antibiotics getting to the injury which therefore would not heal.

I had surgery to my left leg veins similar to the techniques used by heart surgeons. Devices were inserted into the femoral artery and attempts made to clear the blockages. The surgeon was able to clear blockages in the calf but was not able to remove the blockages in my foot. This left me in a precarious situation and may well have dictated the need to have the leg amputated.

I returned home but needed to go back to the hospital because of the pain I was in. Painkilling tablets were insufficient, and I was on morphine which of course is not available to me at home. Whilst in hospital, I underwent a repeat of the surgery in attempt to clear the arteries. This did enable a minor amount of blood to flow but insufficient to fix the problem.

My right leg also shows problems but not as severe as my left. There are likely to be some issues for my heart. I am regularly tested by a heart surgeon and the results have been good, so I am probably OK.

I have named my left leg BILL – Badly Injured Left Leg. Whilst I have suffered injuries to both legs, fractured spinal cords, ribs, arm and facial injuries, the Devil has picked out BILL for special attention. It started in 2008 when I was struck on the inside of the leg just above the ankle by a golf ball. Whilst there was some pain involved, the bruise and swelling which appeared within an hour from my groin to my toes was totally disproportionate to the severity of the impact. I had the injury ultra-scanned to ensure it was OK before catching a flight from Brisbane to Dubai a couple of days later. All seemed well.

However, I suffered a hematoma which basically ate a hole in my leg down to the bone. The skin had not been broken – the problem occurred beneath the surface. It was attended to by a GP in Dubai and appropriately bandaged. I received daily penicillin injections until the danger of infection had passed.

The second incident occurred in 2009 when BILL suffered a deep vein thrombosis (blood clot) which also

Chapter 1 – In Hospital Again

caused pulmonary embolisms on both lungs. This was a life threatening condition but was relatively painless. Fortunately, I realised something was wrong and reported into a hospital emergency ward. The condition was diagnosed very promptly and stabilised. Long term, the peripheral veins needed varicose vein treatment which reduced the fluid retention in the leg, but I have suffered major swelling problems ever since. I also am on blood thinners and am inclined to have clotting should I have to cease the thinners for any reason.

In 2011, I completely ruptured the achilles tendon. Since I was prone to clotting, I was not able to have an operation to repair the damage. I wore a moon boot for several months and it did reattach, but the result was that I was limited to a relatively slow walk. Up until that time I used to compete in runs – City to Surf, half marathons and the like.

In the last few years, I have had problems with both heels – the left worse that the right. The muscle pad, which protects the tibia bone from impact as a step is taken, has atrophied. The was a noticeable recess in both heels. Walking on hard surfaces has been extremely painful. There was also a concern that too much walking could cause stress fractures to the unprotected bone.

And now this latest problem with my arteries. Given the problems I experienced with BILL for many years I don't think my quality of life would change greatly if the lower leg was amputated - it may even improve. Injuries are very hard to heal, and I am prone to infections. The wound left after amputation is a significant challenge. The lower leg needed to be amputated well above the foot to allow space for a prothesis.

An old prayer has provided guidance for me through these difficult times and it goes:-

Lord give me the patience to accept the things I cannot change,
The courage to change the things I can,
And the wisdom to know the difference

Another quote I like is : *Learn to let go of the things you can't change.*

As I cannot change this situation, I accept it. As always, my wife Deborah is very supportive. When she signed up to "in sickness", I don't think she could have contemplated just what would occur. Her support has been an essential element in my journey. In this instance, Deborah helps me with my wheelchair or mobility scooter whenever we go out in the car. She has problems with her back, and it is a severe imposition on her.

So, the leg was amputated. How strange it is to wake up finding your lower leg missing. I cannot believe how effective the pain medication was. I had a tube inserted into my knee reaching down to the wound site close to the major nerves. A pain relief fluid was pumped into my leg at regular intervals, and I had a button to push if the pain got severe, which it rarely did. I also took oral pain killers. Within 3 or 4 days I was on oral pain killers only.

Chapter 1 – In Hospital Again

On day 4 after the operation, I was transferred the Southport Private Rehabilitation Hospital. I immediately was taught how to get out of bed into my wheelchair and back. I set my room up so I could establish an office and move things around as needed.

Within a day I was able to go to the bathroom, shower myself, shave and perform other basic functions. It was bliss to get to this stage after a few days of being confined to bed. I attended physio two times a day. I wheeled myself in the wheelchair to the gym and refused to accept the kind offers of the nurses and physios to push me – I considered the trip was part of my exercise routine. Given it was carpet all the way, my journey was difficult but got easier as I built up strength and got used to the right technique to operate the wheelchair.

I was given an electric scooter by Michelle Miller, a former employee and wife of Don Miller, my best friend and business partner who died in 2021. I think Don is now looking down and very pleased he has been able to help me with the DonMobile.

My prosthesis will not be able to be fitted for a few months, as the wound is very swollen. Initially, the wound was bandaged firmly with stretch bandages to help reduce swelling. Measurements of the knee were taken, and a sock made to be worn all day. Then a temporary prosthesis can be fitted in about two months, and I will be able to walk. About a year later, the wound should be stable and I can get a permanent prosthesis.

Deborah and I have been taught how to get me into and out of a car. That gives me quite a bit of freedom but

I need somebody with me to fold the wheelchair and store it in the car and then unpack it on arrival. A sort of semi-independence but a necessary skill to allow me to live at home and get out and about as necessary. My driving license has been suspended and I need to do a test for it to be reinstated. Equally as important was learning how to stand up to pee which is fundamental to the male psyche.

The physios visited our apartment to see what needed to be done to enable me to grab rails get around. The apartment was refurbished just after my hospitalisation in 2013 and the ensuite is fitted out with grab rails and the like. We had also had a stair lift installed in 2021 when my legs had lost most of their strength. So, the work needed was minimal.

I have been very diligent in maintain an exercise regime all my life. It would be easy to feel cheated by fate, but I choose to appreciate that it is a great benefit to me now.

One of the strangest things that happened was "phantom pain". I got very sharp pains in my missing foot. It occured in several precise locations and will build up sharply before easing. It was impossible to get to sleep when this was happening. Once asleep, it seemed to cease. My sleep varied every night – some nights I was able to get a good night's sleep sometimes, on other nights I would wake at 1:00am and not get any more sleep. I took pain medication, but it didn't fully control the situation. Believe it or not, they recommend you look at the injury when the pain happens, and the pain will cease. Evidently one part of the brain registers that the foot is no longer there and communicates with the part of the brain which registers pain. When I looked

Chapter 1 – In Hospital Again

at the foot, the pain did seem to ease off more quickly. How bizarre! The phantom pain disappeared in a few weeks. As for the amputation injury itself, it gave me little pain.

Whilst the pain went away, I still get feeling in the foot. Sometimes there are pins and needles. I always feel I have a shoe on which is a bit tight. If I try to move the missing foot, it feels like it is encased in plaster which does not allow any movement at all. I have got used to this and whilst the sensation may not go away, I don't see it of concern.

While I was in hospital, there were two physio sessions daily (one on weekends). Since I had always worked out at gyms, I really enjoyed these sessions. The physio session was very well attended, the most common issues being hip or knee surgery. I have a philosophy that I should not wait for inspiration to find me, I need to seek it out. Seeing these mostly elderly people working hard at getting back their mobility does the trick for me. The mood is always positive, and I would like to think I contribute to this comradery.

After the hospital discharge, I became an outpatient of the rehab hospital, attending two days per week. The sessions were longer and more intense than the in-patient sessions.

I did not have any problems occupying my time. Whilst I was in hospital we had the Australian PGA golf, the Australian Open golf, the World Cup (go the Socceroos) and the first two cricket tests Australia V West Indies. I was also working on this book and having a great time recalling the memories (mostly happy) from the past. I also play games on the iPad. In the late afternoon, I had visitors. Deborah saw me daily and various friends and relatives arrive from time to time.

I will now demonstrate what I mean by a finding an inspirational purpose when I was confronted with losing a leg. to which maintains my enthusiasm for life. First, I think of a variety of reasons which could apply:

- I should save 50 % on podiatrist bills. Silly I know but it's worth having a bit of fun even is the issue is serious.
- I still have a life and can function reasonable. True but doesn't inspire me.
- I will be able to maintain my lifestyle which is quite extravagant – pretty good.
- I will lose a few kilos in weight – another silly one.
- A lot have it worse – true but not inspirational.
- I will be walking again by my 70th Birthday. Pretty good as a short-term goal but I want to do better than that.
- I will take up golf again. That really resonates with me. After 40 years of playing golf the pain my left leg when trying to play had become extremely severe and took any enjoyment out of the game. I had reluctantly resigned as a member of the golf club, sold my buggy and given away my clubs.

I figured that if I could manage to play golf again regularly, I would also be able to achieve some other goals such as being able to walks reasonable distances with my dog and swimming in the surf or pool.

When I discussed and agreed the amputation with Vascular Surgeon Venu Bhamidi, I told him I was going to

Chapter 1 – In Hospital Again

play golf again. As it turns out Venu is a friend of friends of mine. He has placed a bet with them that my golf aspirations will be achieved.

I often tell people that I will be playing golf again. Making that verbal commitment increases the chance of success in reaching your goal

And the good thing is if I decide another reason suits me better for a purpose, I am free to use that reason.

I accept the situation I am presented with and will not engage in self-pity. Actually, I did feel a bit sorry for myself, but this was short lived until I got my thinking back to the positive. I refuse to let problems I can't control dictate my feelings and believe this is the key to maintaining my mental health.

Let's face it, I am no stranger to being legless although perhaps in a different context.

I wish to demonstrate in this book that it is possible to perform at a high level despite the multitude of problems Cushing's presents. In fact, the distraction caused by my challenging work took my attention away from my illness. I think this would also apply to those who suffer from any serious health problem. The challenges of my profession and community activities provide a focus for my endeavours which has been very rewarding and has been a great distraction from health concerns which may otherwise have become overwhelming.

And once again I have thwarted the devil!

Chapter 2. Extract from Australian Pituitary Foundation Web Site

The following information relating to Cushing's Disease is provided on the APF web site I am a Director of the APF and thank my fellow board members for their permission to reproduce this fact sheet.

INCIDENCE
Approximately 41 people are diagnosed with Cushing's disease every year in Australia. This represents around 0.16 new cases per 100,000 population per year.

PREVALENCE
Between 300 and 1,600 Australians currently live with Cushing's disease. This represents around 1.2-6.4 cases for every 100,000 population

ABOUT CUSHING'S DISEASE
Cushing's disease is a rare condition that occurs when the body produces too much of the steroid hormone cortisol. This happens as a result of a pituitary tumour producing excessive amounts of the pituitary hormone adrenocorticotropic hormone (ACTH), which in turn stimulates the adrenal glands to produce excessive amounts of cortisol. Cortisol is the main hormone that helps your body deal with stress (such as injury or infection)

and controls blood sugar levels. Occasionally, the ACTH-producing tumour can be located somewhere else in the body. This is referred to as an 'ectopic tumour'.

Cushing's disease specifically refers to the condition of excessive ACTH production by a pituitary tumour. Cushing's syndrome however is the term to describe the condition of excess cortisol in the body which can be due to Cushing's disease or other causes such as long-term use of corticosteroid medication, severe depression, excessive alcohol use or a tumour on the adrenal gland that produces the hormone cortisol.

PRESENTING SIGNS AND SYMPTOMS

Cushing's disease can be difficult to diagnose as some of the symptoms are very common in the general population and occur with other medical conditions. Further, symptoms and signs can develop slowly over long periods of time, making Cushing's disease even harder to recognise.

Physical symptoms
- *Thin, fragile skin that tends to bruise easily*
- *Stretch marks – red/purple streaks across the skin*
- *Muscle loss and weakness*
- *Weight gain, particularly around the waist*
- *Increased fat on back between the shoulders (a 'hump')*
- *Face appears round*
- *Irregular or no menstrual periods (in women)*
- *Hirsutism- excess growth of facial and body hair (in women)*

- *Reduced growth (in children)*
- *Infertility (men and women)*

General symptoms
- *Fatigue*
- *Impaired Quality of Life*
- *Impaired school/work performance*

Emotional Changes
- *Depression*
- *Anxiety*
- *Unable to think clearly*
- *Mood and behavioural changes - personality traits can become more intense*
- *Increased irritability*

Other conditions or complications often seen with Cushing's disease
- Osteoporosis
- Fractures
- High blood pressure
- High blood glucose/Diabetes
- Infections
- Depression

INVESTIGATIONS

No single test is 100% able to diagnose Cushing's disease. Therefore a combination of tests is required which can include:

- *Blood test - to measure hormone levels, including ACTH and cortisol*

- *24-hour urinary free cortisol test - to measure daily cortisol production*
- *Late night or midnight salivary cortisol test - to check for loss of daily cortisol rhythm*
- *Overnight dexamethasone suppression test - to see if cortisol production can be suppressed*
- *Magnetic resonance imaging (MRI) or computed tomography (CT) scan - to see the pituitary gland (and, sometimes, the adrenal gland)*

For some patients, a few other tests are needed including:
- *Inferior petrosal sinus sampling (IPSS) - to check whether ACTH is being released from the pituitary gland or elsewhere*
- *Visual field test - to check for any loss of vision*
- *Bone mineral density (BMD) test - to check bone health.*

If the results indicate Cushing's syndrome rather than Cushing's disease, further tests may be needed to find the source of the high cortisol levels. These are usually organised by an endocrinologist. Around 1 in 6 people (15%) with Cushing's disease have cyclical Cushing's syndrome. This means they rotate between periods of normal and high cortisol production. This means that results can appear normal, depending on when the tests are performed in the cycle. Repeated tests may be necessary to catch a period of high cortisol production.

TREATMENT

The goals of treatment for Cushing's disease are to restore cortisol to normal levels, reverse symptoms and improve quality of life.

This generally requires removing (or controlling the growth of) the pituitary tumour, while maintaining the function of the pituitary gland. Treatment decisions will be tailored to the individual patient, and will depend on a number of features, including the patient's age, gender, the size and location of the pituitary tumour, hormone levels, other medical conditions, current medications, desire for conception, and potential benefits and side effects of treatment. Treatment possibilities include:

1. **Surgery-** *to remove the pituitary tumour. Transsphenoidal surgery is performed in most cases.*
2. **Radiotherapy** - *may be required where surgery is not possible or does not reduce cortisol levels.*
3. **Medication-** *to control cortisol levels.*
4. **Bilateral adrenalectomy** *(removal of the adrenal glands) – used rarely only when surgery and radiotherapy are not possible.*
5. **Medication** *may be used to reduce high cortisol levels before surgery, between surgery and radiotherapy, and/or while waiting for radiotherapy to take effect. Medications fall into three general categories:*
   - **Medications** *that stop the adrenal glands from producing cortisol (ketaconazole, metyrapone, mitotane)*
   - **Medications** *that prevent the pituitary gland from releasing ACTH (cabergoline and pasireotide)*
   - **Medications** *that block the action of cortisol around the body (mifepristone)*

These can be taken alone or in combination.

Chapter 2 – Extract from Australian Pituitary Foundation Web Site

AFTER SURGERY

There are several possible outcomes following surgery.

- *Cortisol levels can remain high (referred to as 'hypercortisolaemia'). If this occurs, repeat surgery or an alternate treatment option will be considered based on individual characteristics.*
- *Cortisol levels can be in a normal range (referred to as 'eucortisolaemia'). If this occurs, your doctor will monitor your cortisol levels as they may change over time.*
- *Cortisol levels can be low (referred to as 'hypocortisolaemia'). Low cortisol levels are the best indication of a successful surgery, as it means the source of increased cortisol had been removed. This requires treatment with cortisol replacement medication (also referred to as steroid therapy). This dose is typically reduced over 6-12 months, however in some cases, cortisol replacement is required longer term. If stopped too early or too quickly, this can have adverse side-effects.*

The hormone changes that occur after a successful surgery can make many patients feel worse and even develop new symptoms, such as nausea, fatigue, depression and anxiety. This is caused by cortisol withdrawal, even if using cortisol replacement medication. Recovery can sometimes take a year or longer. Your doctor should give you written advice about cortisol replacement/steroid therapy and the need to adjust the dose of this medication when stressed or ill.

Wearing a medical alert bracelet/tag and carrying instructions for emergency steroid treatment is essential. It can take months for weight, depression, strength, fatigue and mood to return to normal.

LONG-TERM OUTCOMES

Long-term monitoring is necessary to ensure pituitary function and hormone levels stay in a normal range, and to identify tumour regrowth and/or adjust medication as required. An ongoing concern for those whose Cushing's disease is in remission, is that there is a high rate of recurrence of the condition. For this reason, long-term follow up is strictly required for all people with prior Cushing's disease.

Surgery can result in 'hypopituitarism' — a condition where the pituitary gland is unable to produce other pituitary hormones. If this occurs, long-term hormone replacement therapy will be required.

Radiotherapy may also result in long-term hypopituitarism, which can arise many years after the radiotherapy treatment.

Seeking professional advice and support for management of psychological symptoms is strongly recommended. Following a suitable diet and taking part in regular exercise can help control weight gain.

Chapter 2 – Extract from Australian Pituitary Foundation Web Site

COMMON QUESTIONS

Why am I putting on weight?
Cortisol has many functions in the body, including converting proteins, carbohydrates and fats into energy. If this energy isn't needed, it becomes stored as fat. High levels of cortisol in Cushing's disease can lead to a progressive accumulation of fat.

Why am I so moody?
The excess hormone produced by the tumour has a direct effect on the brain. It tends to produce dramatic mood swings.

Why am I getting facial hair?
The pituitary hormone, ACTH, stimulates the adrenal gland to produce androgens, which promote facial hair growth.

Why do I bruise so easily?
Cortisol increases breakdown of tissue proteins. This causes weakening of the tiny blood vessels near the skin (capillaries), meaning they break easily and cause bruising.

Why have I developed stretch marks?
Cortisol causes increased breakdown of proteins in the skin, which makes the skin more fragile.

Why do I feel so weak?
Too much cortisol causes the increased breakdown of proteins. One effect of this is muscle wasting, which mainly affects muscles in the upper arms and thighs. This can make it difficult to climb stairs or stand after

sitting. Extra weight can also put strain on your muscles, particularly those in your back, sometimes causing back pain and fatigue.

Will I be completely cured after treatment?
In most cases, treatment is successful and usually leads to remission of disease. However, sometimes Cushing's disease can recur. This is why regular follow-up appointments with your endocrinologist are important. Even if you are not cured, most patients find the symptoms improve with treatment.

Is Cushing's disease inherited?
Most cases of Cushing's disease have no inheritance pattern. It has been reported very rarely in families.

Chapter 3. Cushing's Experiences of the Author

My case

The information outlined in Chapter 2 is very applicable to my experience. The following issues are pertinent:

Physical Symptoms
I had all the physical symptoms applicable to a male.

General Symptoms
All applied in my case

Other conditions or complications often seen with Cushing's disease
Applied except for diabetes which thankfully I have not suffered from. I am at the extreme in terms of osteoporosis and resultant bone fractures and muscle weakness causing loss of strength and muscle tears.

Investigations
I underwent all the investigations listed and the cause of my problem is highly likely to be Cushing's Disease. There is a slight doubt which comes about because the MRI scans of my brain do not pick up the tumour. This does occur with some patients and is usually due to the tumour

being very small. There is say a 1% chance that the cause is a tumour elsewhere in my body.

I tell people I have had many brain scans, but they have not found anything.

Treatment
My tumour could not be located which imposed higher risks of damage to the pituitary if surgery was attempted. Drug treatment (Ketoconazole) was prescribed and I was on that drug from 2013 to 2022. At the latter end of that period my physical condition was deteriorating rapidly and I had a bilateral adrenalectomy. By removing the adrenal glands the body can no longer produce cortisol. Early signs are good and hopefully this will improve my health.

Issue not covered
Chapter 2 does not mention the possibility of psychosis, which I did suffer from. I only know a few other sufferers and one of them also suffered from psychosis. Several case studies I have read also involve psychosis and the disease has on some occasions been diagnosed by the attending Psychiatrist.

Hardening of Arteries
I have suffered hardening of arteries. This was first picked upon in 2022 and had obviously been occurring for some. Attempts were made to clear the problem but were unsuccessful. The leg has been amputated below the knee. Scans show the blood flow in the right leg is poor. The arteries around the heart require checking as well.

Time to Diagnose and Morbidity

Cushing's is a life threatening disease particularly if not treated. There seems to be a morbidity rate of 50% in 5 years. It is difficult to determine when that 5 year periods starts. Most of us who suffer from Cushing's have the disease suffer for many years prior to diagnosis. In my case I would have suffered for about ten years with all the physical symptoms in place for 5 years. I would not have lived much longer.

A Not So Rare Disease

Given the combination of extensive delays in diagnosis and high morbidity rates, it is inevitable that a significant number of people are dying without being diagnosed.

Chapter 4. My Father

My father Morgan John (Jack) O'Brien was the most significant role model in my life. He was a gentle and highly intelligent man who led a very hard life both financially and from a health perspective.

His mother Laura died in 1918 when he was only 8 years old, leaving him and his sister Lorna with different members of her family. His father (also Morgan John) was not involved in Dad's upbringing from that point. It is not clear whether they were estranged prior to her death. He was referred to as "that bloody Irishman" by his in laws and was obviously unpopular with them. I have done some family history research which reveals some unsavoury incidents in his life – nothing criminal but deeds of which he couldn't have been proud.

One of the stories Jack did tell was that his father turned up at the door many years after Laura's death, but Jack refused to see him.

Laura's family were from the Southwest of England and their religions were Baptist, Methodist and the like. As she married Morgan Snr in a Catholic Church in Adelaide, I can only assume she converted to Catholicism prior to the wedding.

Chapter 4 – My Father

Jack was sent to a Catholic boarding school in Adelaide and spent the holidays with his uncle and aunt (Bert and Gert) at Mt Lofty in the Adelaide Hills where Bert was a gardener.

Jack was obviously not happy at the school. He refused to take confirmation as required by the Church and was caned several times but would not give in. He was always highly principled and such behaviour was consistent with an injustice having been done. What that was is not known. When Jack was in his elder years, he was befriended by a Catholic Priest He refused to reconcile with the church but maintained the friendship with the Priest.

He did well at school, to the extent that at the end of his 10th year he was offered a cadetship in Journalism. Within him there was a love of the English language which was to remain with him for life. His uncle and aunt determined that journalism was not a proper job, and that he should take up a trade.

He took up an apprenticeship as a painter which was completed in 1929. If you were to name the most undesirable occupations in the great depression, I am sure that painting would be near the top of the list. People did without things being painted or did it themselves.

At that time Jack became homeless. He rarely talked about this. One story he did tell was that he was fortunate enough one day to find a couple of onions. He commenced cooking them but was too hungry to wait, so "ate the bloody things raw". He also did tell us he carried the "waltzing matilda (swag) for a while.

The depression continued up until the start of World War 2. Like so many others Jack volunteered for the army and was trained in the 2/48 Rifle Battalion, in South Australia. For the first time he was earning a regular salary.

He was transferred to the Middle East where he was given training as a Morse code operator. Why would be selected for such training? I suspect he was observed doing his Times Cryptic Crosswords which he did daily for his whole life. Such a skill was considered a great qualification for both Morse code and code breaking. Misinterpretation of the dots, dashes and spaces resulted in corrupted messages, and someone had to interpret what was really meant.

The 2/48 Rifle Battalion saw action during the siege of Tobruk and the Second Battle of El Alamein. Dad never spoke of this. Clearly, he did his training for signals whilst in the Middle East, but I do not know what action he was involved in.

Following the Japanese attack on Pearl Harbour and subsequent push to Papua New Guinea, Jack was amongst the many Australian Troops recalled for service in PNG.

For those who don't know the history of Australia's troops from returning from the Middle East, it was because of the determination of our newly elected Prime Minister John Curtin who recognised the threat to Australia presented by the Japanese and the need to align ourselves with America. Winston Churchill thought that the "Dominion" troops should be under the control of Britain. He opposed the return of the Australians and stated the Japanese would

Chapter 4 – My Father

not be able to take "Fortress Singapore" – as it turned out they did take it after a battle which only took 3 days.

Curtin was adamant and the troops were returned. Churchill had another try at regaining control of the Australian Troops when he ordered two of the ships carrying troops back to Australia to be diverted to Rangoon (now Yangon) in Burma (now Myanmar). The Japanese were building up for an attack on Burma and Churchill was desperate to hold them back. Curtin heard of this and countermanded the orders. Given the lack of preparedness of the Australian troops their involvement would have been futile. Jack was on board one of the troop carriers and I doubt many Australians would have survived had Churchill had his way. Dad was on one of those vessels and had Churchill succeeded in diverting then to Rangoon I doubt very much that he would have survived.

I won't go into the details of Jack's service in PNG but will provide some of the more amusing tales he told. As with most of our returned servicemen he rarely spoke of the more harrowing aspects of the war. However, no one should doubt the brutality of the war in PNG and the effect it had on our troops.

Before regaling you with those tales, I should make you aware that Jack suffered from Coeliac Disease. The disease was not discovered until the 1950s. The diet in the army was far from gluten free and he continually suffered from intestinal problems. He also contracted malaria which recurred for the rest of his life. Add to that the dysentery suffered by all troops in that campaign – how horrific that must have been.

He was very grateful to a Salvation Army Chaplain he came to know. The Chaplain used to "liberate" tobacco, alcohol and food from the Americans and "reassign" them to the Aussies and KIWIS. A modern Robin Hood. I suspect the Americans were willing to look the other way as this occurred.

One of his responsibilities was to repair cut communications cables. To do so, both hands were needed to feel for the break. The rifle had to be slung over the shoulder. Jack was in this situation when he saw a Japanese soldier staring at him, gun in hand. They both let out a startled yell, turned around and ran in opposite directions.

After the end of the war, the army relocated Jack to Brisbane. He went to a dance at the Camp Hill School of Arts where he met Peggy who had 3 children and a failed marriage. Peggy was living in the family home which was nearby.

It was a match made in heaven. Of course, at that point in time divorce was shameful, so they moved to Adelaide along with Peggy's daughters Desley and Jeanette. The eldest child Frank remained with his father in Brisbane. That must have been devastating for Peggy.

Chapter 5. My Mother

Mum was borne Florence Rose James but known from early childhood as Peggy. Evidently my Uncle Alf would sit her on his knee and sing a song about Peggy to her and that became her name.

Her father George was a very small man and was never healthy enough to work, the family surviving on a pension. The house in Camp Hill was a very basic workers cottage which was constructed in about 1920 using mainly secondhand timber from the Coorparoo racetrack which was being demolished at the time.

George's lack of employment provided ample opportunity for other endeavours and he and Maggie had 7 children. How they fitted into the house beggars belief.

Peggy's older siblings started attending Camp Hill Primary School on the opening day of 1 July 1926 which started life as the Mt Bruce School, that being to previous name of the suburb of Camp Hill. She started school a year or two later. Since then, the extended James family have been very prominent at the school.

Mum was very knowledgeable on the history of Camp Hill. She would point out the route for the Belmont Flyer which was an early example of private rail. Up to 1910, the Council unsuccessfully lobbied for a rail line to the area. The council eventually borrowed funds and built a railway line from Norman Park Station, through Seven Hills and Carina to Belmont. The Belmont Flyer line opened in 1912 but closed in 1924 due to non-profitability. The line reopened briefly in 1926.

Later a tram line was built I several stages which provided a connection from the City to Carina. It was always called the Belmont tram even though it stopped several kms short of Belmont, presumably because the final stage was never completed. It ceased operation in the late 1960s.

Peggy fell pregnant at 16 yrs old and "had to marry". Frank Jnr was duly born, and she and Frank Snr had two daughters, Desley and Jeanette. The marriage was a disaster and the couple separated.

She went to a dance at the local Camp Hill School of Arts where she met Jack. They quicky became a couple.

Chapter 6. My upbringing

In 1946, it was a matter of great shame for my mother to separate from her husband, let alone to become involved with another man. Jack and Peggy must have felt unwanted in such an environment and, together with Desley and Jeanette they moved to the Adelaide suburb of Payneham, a short distance from where Jack had spent his early childhood. They lived in a ramshackle cottage. Frank Jnr was left with his father which no doubt was a heartbreaking decision for Peggy.

They found acceptance from his mother's family and life started getting better. Jack worked at a range of occupations including painting where he had served his apprenticeship. He had some very bad falls which resulted in major back injuries. Along with that, the Malaria suffered in Papua New Guinea recurred every time he caught a cold. And the yet to be diagnosed Coeliac disease caused distress from time to time. This trio of maladies would cause him problems for the remainder of his life.

Other occupations included working as a truck driver on the construction of the Maralinga site which was used by the British for testing nuclear weapons and also a stint as a taxi driver. Given his lack of employment in the depression years, he was willing to take on any job and go wherever needed to support his family.

Jack accepted Desley and Jeanette as his own children as they accepted him as their father. There were none of the strains expected in a stepfather/stepdaughter relationship. After many years of hardship and loneliness, he found himself in a loving family.

Desley had some sort of handicap which I don't think was ever diagnosed – not unusual in those days. She was a very gentle and loving sole and a wonderful sister to me. Jeanette was rowdy and boisterous, the life of the party. Always fun to be with.

In 1946, along came Raelene. What a joy that must have been for Jack and Peg!

The family moved to Blair Athol in Adelaide, and I was born in 1953. Once again, the "house" was a rented cottage. A boy baby must have been a blessing to them. Particularly one as cute as me!

Back in Brisbane, Peggy's father, George, was in a very poor state of health. Maggie (George's wife) was also unwell, suffering from dementia. In 1956, Jack and Peggy agreed to move into her family home in Camp Hill, Brisbane to care for them. Our family packed up and hopped on the train for the trip. Unfortunately, George died before we arrived in Brisbane.

The cottage was cosy to say the least. Jack and Peggy in the main bedroom, Maggie in the sleep out (old verandah) and the four kids in double bunks in the one bedroom. Whilst Camp Hill has these days changed into a trendy suburb, it was very much a working-class suburb then.

Chapter 6 – My upbringing

Maggie was the only grandparent I met, and I never felt accepted by her. Neither did my sister Raelene. This could have been due to Maggie's misgivings about Peggy's divorce. It may also have been due to her dementia. Walking to the bus stop naked in the early morning seemed to indicate not all was well.

School for us was Camp Hill Infants, and Camp Hill Primary, following the footsteps of Peggy and her siblings, the James family. I generally attended bare footed. Before school and in the breaks, we would play cricket, rugby league, soccer or British Bulldog on the oval. This required considerable courage and tolerance to pain as there wasn't a blade of grass on the oval. There was an abundance of rocks and a concrete cricket pitch.

I was often required to go to the corner shop to pick up an item or 2 of groceries. Mum gave me a note which always included 3 pence of lollies for Dennis. On more than one occasion I came home with the lollies and forgot the groceries. Choosing lollies was great. The whole selection sat in a drawer of about 1200 x 800 and 100 high with a glass top. You pointed out the lollies you want, and these were added to a white paper bag. The best were rockets, a chocolate coated piece of licorice which at 8 per penny represented the best value. Milk bottles and raspberries were good but at only 3 per penny were a tad expensive.

My trip to the shop took me past the home of Mr and Mrs Day. They were from Days dairy which was quite big farm in the 19th century and their house occupied a very small part of the old farm. Mr Day was blind, and I only occasionally saw him. Mrs Day was a very nice lady who used to spend a lot of time in the garden and mowing, those tasks falling upon her. They had two daschunds which in true daschund style always bounded out barking at me before submitting to a pat. Mrs Day would always have a chat to me and was a lovely lady and I hope my impatience to get to the shop for my lollies was not too apparent.

Academically I was near the top of the class, with a particular bent towards mathematics. My English was pretty good – having a father who loved the language stood me in good stead then and remains the case now. I enjoyed history and geography. Then there were the artistic subjects – drama, art, technical drawing. My work was crap, and I have maintained this level of performance in artistic endeavours my entire life.

During this time my father worked mainly in paint sales, being a technical representative for various paint manufacturers. This included travelling throughout Northern New South Wales visiting hardware shops. In 1960 there was a very sharp recession and Jack was dismissed. Our Prime Minister Robert Menzies called an election which he won by one seat, our local seat of Belmont which was won narrowly by Jim Killen for the Liberal Party. This prompted the famous telegram from Menzies "Killen you are magnificent". In later years Jim would enjoy a comradery with Geoff Whitlam and Fred Daly despite them being famous Labour figures.

Chapter 6 – My upbringing

Jack managed to get a part time job delivering milk. He would spend each evening in absolute agony with his back. He then managed to get a job managing the paint in a hardware in Armidale – he had known the owners from his days as a travelling salesman. He would visit home every month or so and I can recall being distraught when he left.

Meanwhile Peggy also worked to help make ends meet and to provide some money leading up to Jack's retirement. She was the school cleaner at Camp Hill Infants School for many years. I used to earn a little pocket money helping her in the afternoons. She also worked as a cleaner in various households. Another role was in Myers at Coorparoo where she worked at the chicken counter.

She also had a large workload at home looking after her 4 children and Jack. She did this cheerfully and was always singing very tunefully. The song I remember most was The Gypsy Rover which also has some whistling which she handled well. It is on an Irish Rovers album in my music collection and brings a tear to my eye every time I play it.

Our meals were simple "meat and 2 veg". Sundays called for a special lunch. One of our chickens would be ritually beheaded, plucked and hung up to bleed before Peggy would roast it along with potatoes. Jack had a vegetable garden with a variety of vegies always available. His favourite was broad beans. He would put the water on to boil, then pick the broad beans. It doesn't come any fresher than that.

Meals stepped up a notch on the purchase of out "tucker box freezer". These were the first domestic freezer sold and were a real status symbol. Now we could buy a whole rump or side of lamb and carve it into meal size proportions before freezing it for future consumption.

I was allowed a lot of freedom at a very young age. Often on Saturday, I would walk up to the Planet Cinema in Camp Hill to see the matinee. Usually, it was a cartoon followed by a western. The cost? One shilling and sixpence (15 cents) for entry and another sixpence for an ice cream or a packet of Jaffas – two bob (20 cents) in total. The Jaffas were perfect for rolling down the timber aisles and making a racket.

Another treat was to catch the tram to the Gabba after school to see the last session of a Sheffield Shield match. Entry was free after the tea break. This was financed by collecting bottles and returning these to the canteen. One of the grandstands had tiered timber flooring and seats but no vertical upstand. My mates and I would walk in under the stand and reach though to vertical opening to grab the bottle which was not necessarily fully empty. Normally we made more in bottle collections that we spent on tram rides and refreshments.

For many years I was not allowed to have a radio. We wasn't one in the house. I think my parents didn't want me listening to the radio instead of studying. As I did little in the way of study, this obviously didn't help at all. Dad's car however did have a radio. I can remember 4:00 am when I would go down to the car with the keys, turn the ignition on and listen to the cricket from the West Indies. Simpson, Lawry and co against Wes Hall and Gary Sobers, with Alan MacGilvray commentating.

Chapter 6 – My upbringing

When my parents gave a little ground, I was given a Crystal Radio. It was a clear plastic device the shape of an egg. Incoming signal was via 2 leads which clipped onto whatever steel wires were available. The Hills hoist rotary clothes line was the quintessential Aussie crystal antenna. Output was a very weak signal to a single earpiece.

A couple of years later I was given an Astor transistor radio and really hit the big time. Then I purchased a record player for myself and started collecting my own records.

Favourite activities after school and on weekends were cricket, touch football, and cowboys and "itchybums" with other kids on the street. Cricket was played on the bitumen road. Occasionally a car would come along, and we would move the stumps (garbage bins) aside to let the car through.

At the ripe old age of 9 I commenced playing rugby league with Eastern suburbs. My first few trial matches were in the under fourteens which put me at considerable size and weight disadvantage. Also in the side those few weeks was Paul Khan who I became friendly with. He sold me a pair of secondhand boots for 1 pound. Paul was a couple of years older than me and was a star throughout his junior career and ended up plying quite a few tests for Australia.

The boots he sold me were crap. In those days football boots resembled work boots with tags on the soles. I wore blisters on my heels every training session and game and they always burst and bled. Our coach had a ready-made cure for this. "Piss in a bucket and put it on your heels.

That'll harden the buggers up"". I did this and it seemed to work, although the potential for infection was probably extreme and I certainly would not recommend it. As it turned out, I had spurs on my heels when I was young and that was the cause of my problem. Dad took me to a surgical bootmaker, and I was provided with a set of handmade boots made from kangaroo leather which was very light and soft. A couple of years later Adidas came out with their boots which I was able to use straight off the shelf. They were available only in manly black with the three white stripes – none of these orange and green fairy slippers worn by current players.

Fences were few and dogs many. When was the last time you saw a dog chase a car? What would they have done if they ever caught one?

The most spectacular event in this period of my life was the fire at the Camp Hill State School. It was a Saturday afternoon, and I was walking home from a friend's place when I saw the smoke and fire. I raced home the rest of the way, ran up the front stairs yelling "The schools on fire". Then out the back door and up the road to the school. The wing affected was parallel to the main road, Old Cleveland Road, and included my classroom. Students lined up along the opposite side of the road. Each time a roof or wall collapsed, the class who occupied the room cheered. Class 6C certainly was one of the rowdiest.

My education took me to Camp Hill High School. At that point, I needed to select my subjects and, having some talent in the maths area, I went into the maths and

Chapter 6 – My upbringing

sciences stream. I managed to stay near the top of the class but did not put in a major effort.

I remember vividly the 14th of February 1966, the day Australia introduced decimal currency. The advertising jingle was "Clink go the cents boys, clink, clink, clink" sung to the music of "Click go the shears". We had one dollar and two dollar notes, one and two cent coins, and a 12-sided 50 cent piece, all of which are now defunct.

I continued with my favourite sports of Rugby League and Cricket, where I enjoyed a reasonable amount of success, but it was clear I would need to concentrate on my academic

future. In grade 11, there was a scholarship exam held. I was one of the few at Camp Hill who was awarded a scholarship. It was an IQ based test and it was at that time I started to consider that I might have the talent to attend University and study Engineering.

The driving force for me was my father. Here was a highly intelligent man who spent much of his life in poverty, due to bad luck and lack of opportunity. There was no way I would let an opportunity pass me by. That attitude remains with me to this day.

The other thing I have inherited is a fear of losing wealth through economic circumstances. I have been reasonably successful financially but have been cautious not to "bet the farm" on any investment. I shall call it my "Inherited Depression Syndrome".

For some strange reason I grew up thinking women were weak and needed my protection. Maybe it was my grandmother's frail state. Somehow, I thought my mother was weak – how strange given the way she handled herself with her young children and worked most of her life in an era where the wife stayed at home and looked after the kids. That misconception caused me to make very poor judgements in later life.

We had next door neighbors who built on the last allotment in our area. Until the late 50's the block had been the last remnants of a creek. I can remember having a great time sliding down the piles of cinders which were delivered to fill in the creek bed. It cost me some scratches and a lot of black dirt which needed to be washed off.

Our neighbours moved in – husband and wife, two sons about my age and a daughter a little younger. I spent a lot of time playing cricket next door. Often at night we would hear the father abusing his wife and I have no doubt the domestic violence was at an extreme level. One afternoon the younger son told me "Mummy's gone to sleep in the toilet". I was only 6 at the time and went with him to see. Sure enough, there she was on the toilet floor. I was not old enough to realise she had died.

After that there were a series of "housemaids" who were verbally abused and probably physically abused as well. The language used was appalling. Alter a few years the father remarried a lady - "Pixie". She was able to notice the signs when her husband was heading towards an abusive state – a bottle or two of rum was a bit of a

Chapter 6 – My upbringing

giveaway. She would leave the house and come into our place where my parents and I would sit and talk to her. After a while she would judge when her husband would have fallen asleep and return home. Her being in our house at these times caused me concern – I could imagine her husband running amuck. But I thought if my parents were showing such kindness, then so should I.

And why did Pixie put up with it? Because of concern for his children.

I had a series of part time jobs. The first one was work in a café during the Brisbane Exhibition (the Ecca), which I did every year from age 12 to 17.

I used to work on Saturday washing trucks for Cavanagh Bros at Milton. On completion of high school, I worked at a factory which made 44-gallon drums whilst awaiting exam results and job applications. It was very physical work in hot conditions and the wages were $22 per week including overtime. It certainly made me focus on finding a role in engineering.

My father managed paint departments for various hardware stores in my high school years and he managed to get me a job as a storeman in the weeks leading up to Christmas. I saved a considerable amount from my earnings from my part time jobs and the scholarship which my parents insisted I keep for my education.

Just before Christmas in 1970, a huge hailstorm hit the southern suburbs. I was working at a hardware with my father, and we were subjected to hail the size of golf balls, which smashed through roof panels in the hardware. My sister Raelene and her husband Barry had a house in Woodridge with a steel roof. The steel was split and had to be replaced. People with fibro rooves had to sit under tables - the hail smashed through the roof and the ceiling and landed on the floor below.

Amongst the devastation, Jack came up with an opportunity. Firstly, he got on the phone and ordered every tin of blackjack and roll of bituminous paper available in Brisbane (both used for temporary repair of rooves). I got the task of cutting the bituminous paper into 1 M strips which kept me busy for a couple of days. People were queued down the street waiting to get their tar and paper. It was the only hardware store in the area which had these materials.

During these years, I also increasingly took on a lot of the physical work required by the family. Jack's poor physical condition made it difficult for him, but he still insisted on doing his share. He would then spend hours in great agony. By age 12 I could put up our tent (a very heavy George Pickers 15 ft x 15ft). First the corner posts, pegs and ropes. Then the centre pole, followed by the 8 side posts, pegs and ropes. Then redoing the pegs and ropes so that everything was square. Then came 2 additional poles pegs and ropes to allow the front of the tent to act as an annex. Next was a trench around the perimeter of the tent to slow the ingress of water during the inevitable summer storms.

Before I took on this work, Jack would have to do it with some help. A highlight for us every year was when he

Chapter 6 – My upbringing

always kicked a tent peg and, on several occasions, I am sure he broke a toe. Whilst he groaned in agony, the rest of the family laughed hysterically - "the silly old bugger's done it again". It was no use expecting sympathy from the O'Brien tribe.

I mowed the yard. When the house needed painting, I took on the task. Sewerage came to us, and I dug the trenches for the pipework.

In 1979, Jack became seriously ill and lost a large amount of weight. We all thought he had a cancer. He was in hospital for several weeks and was diagnosed with coeliac disease. He changed to a gluten free diet and immediately regained the lost weight. We had to be very careful with his food at that critical stage as the tiniest amount of gluten would make him very ill.

He made a claim against the army for illnesses suffered during the war. The army knocked the claim back, but Jack was determined that he should receive a veteran's pension which would also continue be paid to Peggy after his death. He appealed against the decision. Whilst he was entitled to have a solicitor to represent him, there was no money available for that. He represented himself and won the case. This, together with the hard work of both my parents put them in a reasonable, but far from extravagant situation in retirement.

I look at the current situation where our returned service people suffer from PTSD and the Defence forces avoid dealing with it and wonder whether anything has changed.

Jack went to extraordinary lengths to help people who were doing it tough. No doubt his memories of the depression years were etched permanently in his mind. He was one of the locals at the Camp Hill Hotel which until the 60's was a magnificent old Queenslander. Unfortunately, it was pulled down and replaced with an eyesore.

I would sometimes get to go with him in the afternoon and sit on the verandah with my raspberry lemonade. Jack would be in the public bar (complete with sawdust floor) with mates. It would be quite common for him to arrive home with a stranger he met who was having a tough time. Peggy would cook a bit extra that night. That was the time of the 6 O'Clock close which limited his opportunity to consume too much XXXX.

One night he arrived home with a work mate, George Gilbert, a.k.a. Pommy George. I think George was of Indian or Pakistani descent, but such distinctions meant nothing to us. His accent was English, and I assume he had lived in England all his life. His wife and young daughters had been killed in a railway derailment. He left for Australia to start a new life.

George had nowhere to stay, so he slept on a mattress on the floor that night and for several months thereafter until he could find his own accommodation in an adjoining property to ours.

George was particularly fond of my sister Raelene who no doubt evoked memories of his daughters. He was also very generous to me. Our favourite pastime was crab fishing. George would hire a rowboat and we would head out from Wellington Point to catch sand crabs. On other occasions, we would try our luck with mud crabs in a creek. Our enthusiasm greatly exceeded our expertise, and we rarely had a worthwhile catch.

He once took me out shooting and after some practice at dawn, a wallaby stood on the side of the road. I was given the task of shooting it, aimed carefully and shot it through the throat. On the one hand I was proud of the shot. On the other I was appalled at having destroyed a life. I have never attempted to harm an animal since that day.

George remained a close friend of the family until he died in the 1990's.

Chapter 7. Cadetship 1971 to 1977

Having achieved a sufficient result in my Year 12 exams in 1970, it was time to consider how I would achieve my goal of an engineering degree. I really was quite ignorant of the range of specialisations involved. No one in my family and circle of friends was an engineer. I knew engineers designed bridges and that sounded pretty cool. I knew that the type of engineer who designed bridges was a civil engineer. I would become a civil engineer!

Two other factors weighed heavily on my planning. My parents were approaching retirement age and had only recently been in a situation where they could accumulate a modest amount of wealth. It was time for me to cease being a financial burden on them.

The second issue was that while still at High School I had met Margaret. We were determined to get married. I needed an income to support her.

The Queensland Railway Department advertised scholarships in Civil Engineering offering scholarships to attend Queensland University for four years with a modest stipend. Engineering Degrees require the student to work for an appropriate employer each year for practical experience. QR provided that

Chapter 7 – Cadetship 1971 to 1977

holiday employment. After interviews and due consideration, I was offered a position.

Meanwhile I had applied for a cadetship in Mechanical Engineering with the State Department of Works. My education would be via a part time course at the Queensland Institute of Technology (now called the Queensland University of Technology). I would be employed full time, with time off to attend lectures. A weekly schedule would involve two evening lectures and two afternoon lectures for six years assuming I did not fail any subjects. My work as a Mechanical Engineer would include designing Air Conditioning Systems.

The position with State Works suited me better and I accepted, thinking I could transfer to Civil Engineering in the first few years, when the courses were identical. Regarding the railway position, I find it remarkable that at the end of my career, I found myself responsible for a group of railway consultants.

On my first day with State Works, I was given the standard specifications to read. I remember reading the standard spec for ductwork. I didn't know what a duct was. I was provided with the Carrier Design Manual (William Carrier was the inventor of air conditioning). It was way beyond my level of comprehension. It took a long time for me to develop an understanding of the theories involved.

I had some practical training in the department's workshop. I learned such diverse things as repairing fans and chemically treating a swimming pool.

The Department carried out some design in-house, with other work being let to consulting engineers. The in-house projects were generally smaller projects which were often unusual. It was the era of the Bjelke-Peterson Government and there was no shortage of funds for Department of Primary Industry projects. I also worked on some interesting projects in prisons and institutions. This provided a diverse range of experience which included:
- A research piggery
- Kitchens and laundries.
- Plant growth cabinets
- A dairy
- An artificial insemination centre for export of cattle semen.

One job I remember in particular was a methyl bromide fumigation facility and the insights into occupational health and safety in a bygone era. Like all other States, Queensland has strict laws on what plant matter (i.e. fruit, vegetables and flowers) can be brought in from overseas or other states. I was required to design a facility where this could be done with minimal risk to the workers. Much later in my career I wrote an OH & S system for NDY, and I will attempt to write a procedure for the fumigation as it existed in the 70s, perhaps tainted by my sense of the absurd.

Procedure for Methyl Bromide Fumigation

Equipment:
- *One tank of methyl bromide gas with valve, hose, and spray nozzle*
- *A bloody big tarpaulin*

Chapter 7 – Cadetship 1971 to 1977

Procedure:

1. *Identify site which can be cleared of people. One person to be available to ensure no people are near the fumigation for the entire duration of the work.*
2. *Identify wind direction.*
3. *Ensure fruit, veggies and flowers are in well ventilated containers. Place them in the site as identified above.*
4. *Place the tarpaulin over the fruit veggies and flowers.*
5. *Place the methyl bromide canister next to the tarpaulin.*
6. *Take a really big breath and hold it.*
7. *Open the valve, lift an edge of the tarpaulin, and spray the methyl bromide onto the fruit, veggies and flowers.*
8. *Run like buggery upwind to a safe distance.*
9. *Exhale and then continue normal breathing.*
10. *Wait for 5 mins.*
11. *Take a really big breath and hold it.*
12. *Run to the tarpaulin and remove it.*
13. *Run like buggery upwind to a safe distance.*
14. *Exhale and then continue normal breathing.*
15. *Wait for 5 mins.*
16. *Pack up the fruit, veggies and flowers*
17. *Procedure complete.*

Whist this has a funny side to it, it did put workers at considerable risk and highlights just how far we have come in terms of workplace safety.

I also handled a multitude of commercial air conditioning projects which provided the basis for my future work.

Toward the end of my cadetship, I was transferred to the Project Liaison Group where I was responsible for:
- Monitoring upcoming projects
- Liaising with inhouse groups to determine whether the project would be carried out inhouse or by an external consulting firm.
- For external projects, preparing a brief
- Keeping record of the work given to each consultant.
- Suggesting an appropriate consultant for each project
- Conducting a briefing meeting for the external consultant which included the project architect and others as appropriate.

This proved invaluable to me as I established contact with senior representatives of most of the engineering consulting practices and architectural firms in Brisbane.

Meanwhile, I married Margaret in 1972 at the ripe old age of 19. Our first born was Belinda in 1974. In that year we purchased some land and had a house constructed. We were able to do this thanks to a favourable loan available through the Public Service and our own savings. Neither of our families were in a position to offer financial assistance, nor would we have sought such assistance.

In the first 4 years of my cadetship, there was little time for sport, and I did insufficient exercise, which resulted in significant weight gain. I went back to playing rugby league in the public service competition for two years and got myself back into reasonable shape.

Chapter 7 – Cadetship 1971 to 1977

My final exams were in 1976. I managed to get through the course without failing or deferring a subject which was rare for a part time student. I decided to seek employment with a Consulting Practice, and I applied for positions with two very good firms who I had worked with in my role with the Project Liaison Group and both offered me a position.

I accepted a role with Norman Disney & Young. Russell Brothers was the Queensland Director, and we knew each other from previous projects. I had reviewed documents prepared by NDY and thought them to be superior to any of the other practices. The company only had 8 staff in Brisbane, having only started a Brisbane office a few years earlier. They had established offices in Sydney, Melbourne and Perth. I thought they would be likely to grow and provide opportunities for me. That turned out to be a great choice.

The process of obtaining this employment left me with an insight for future years when I was the one employing staff. Good staff are hard to find and have their choice of employers. Success in employing staff requires the employer to sell the firm to the applicant.

Chapter 8. NDY Queensland 1977 to 1987

I found myself surrounded by very competent people. As founding director, David Norman had a very focussed approach to the business of Consulting Engineering. This summarises some of the key events behind the success of the company.

David studied for his Degree in Mechanical Engineering in the early 1950's. One of his vacation employment opportunities was at the Woomera Rocket Range. Some of the facilities had air conditioning, which was only invented in 1937 and was rare in Australia.

He foresaw that air conditioning would be a great growth industry in Australia. He then turned his mind to how he could acquire the necessary expertise to be a major player. At that time, Carrier Air Conditioning were the leaders in the field. David could not get a green card to enable him to work in USA with Carrier. He did the next best thing and applied for a job with Carrier in Canada. He was successful.

Within a couple of years, David was Chief Design Engineer for Carrier Canada. Not only did he learn how to design air conditioning systems, but he also acquired skills in managing a technology-based business.

Chapter 8 – NDY Queensland. 1977 to 1987

In 1959, HD Norman and Associates was established in North Sydney. The firm became Norman and Addicoat and then Norman Disney & Young in 1969.

David was passionate about minimising energy use and established the company's reputation on low energy systems. At that time, scant regard was paid to energy efficiency due in part to the very low cost of energy in Australia. David built up a formidable team of Mechanical Engineers is Sydney. Branches were set up throughout Australia and were able to tap into the Sydney expertise in Air Conditioning. They were also instrumantal in growing the firm in other areas of Building Services – Electrical, Lifts, Fire Services, Hydraulics, Acoustics and Communications.

David's business model was based on the following principals
- Knowledge acquired on projects would be shared across the organisation. This was achieved by establishing documentation systems and design guidelines which were available to all employees
- Employing young talented staff and providing them with opportunities for advancement.
- Establishing a culture whereby sharing of expertise was the norm.

And so, I found myself surrounded by people who were committed to my career development. Not only was I able to seek assistance from the two very experienced Mechanical Engineers in Brisbane, I was able to tap into the vast pool of knowledge in other offices.

I learnt a great deal from the drafters in the office. At that time nobody had contemplated computer aided drafting – this was all ink pens, tracing film and handwritten notes. When a mistake was made, out came the razor blade. It was very important to get it right first time. The drafters taught me the basics and helped me to focus on the practical side of things.

A similar situation occurred with typing which was done by an electric typewriter directly onto paper. It was then photocopied through a Xerox Machine to provide multiple copies.

I small mistake could be corrected by a little liquid paper. A larger error could cause a great deal of retyping.

Photocopying could be a dangerous pastime. The copying machines of that era needed heaters to dry the ink. If a paper jam occurred, a fire was likely. So a copier always had to be attended so that any paper jam could be dealt with.

I was entrusted with an increasing complexity of projects. Where NDY was appointed for several different disciplines, a Project Coordinator was appointed. I was appointed as PC on some projects. And so my skills expanded.

I remember learning a valuable lesson in client relationships. I was PC on a project where the Architect would have preferred another consultant. I was very diligent and made sure all my tasks were completed. The Electrical Engineer was Bob Cushway, an Associate of NDY. Bob had a very relaxed attitude to deadlines during

Chapter 8 – NDY Queensland. 1977 to 1987

the design but at the end of the design period put in the hours necessary to get a good job out on time. At one project meeting Bob was asked if had done the sketch of a special light fitting.

Bobs' answer was "I was going to say that I had the sketch done but the print machine broke down. But you would know that I was bullshitting, so I haven't done it." This was met with laughter and there was no problem. Meanwhile I was doing everything I was asked to and copping criticism. The lesson for me was to lighten up and show a sense of humour.

During my time in Brisbane, I did little exercise and my fitness suffered accordingly.

In 1979, NDY was appointed for Paradise Centre, a full city block in the centre of Surfer's Paradise. Well known hotelier and developer Eddie Kornhauser had a vision which included an international hotel, two apartment towers, shopping centre, entertainment centre and Surf Life Saving Club.

Our Brisbane office was overloaded at the time. NDY Perth provided the staff to get the job to schematic design phase.

I was offered a transfer to the Gold Coast to handle the Mechanical Services. Another colleague was to handle electrical services. A year later my colleague returned to Brisbane, and I took on the role as Gold Coast Manager. To put this in context, I was a 26 year old engineer being entrusted to run the Building Services on Australia's largest commercial project at the time. It was a stunning opportunity and I often reflect on how difficult that decision must have been for the NDY Directors.

Don Miller was to become the Electrical Engineer for the office. Don and I were the best of mates until he died in 2021.

We had major problems obtaining staff at in the 1980s. There was no university on the Gold Coast at that time and the local economy was (and still is) subject to major booms and busts. It was difficult to attract employees. The first few years we were understaffed, and the workload was formidable. Nonetheless we enjoyed ourselves immensely and the profits were excellent mainly because you don't pay staff you don't have. We took on engineers and drafters with limited experience who were willing to give it a go and we were able to train them in relatively quick time.

Margaret and I had Jodie in 1977 and Danielle came along in 1979. We moved home to Waterford which was halfway between Brisbane and the Gold Coast

Working on Paradise Centre proved a unique experience and I have had lifelong friendships with many people from that team – Architects, Builders, other Engineers, Quantity Surveyors and Project Managers. I still meet for lunch with several of them on a regular basis.

To ensure the continued success of the Gold Coast Office, we needed to obtain further work and we were very successful in that regard. Projects won included Holiday Inn Surfer's Paradise, Sanctuary Cove, expansion of Pacific Fair Shopping Centre, Sheraton Mirage Main Beach, and

Chapter 8 – NDY Queensland. 1977 to 1987

Marina Mirage Main Beach. In recognition of this I was promoted to the level of Associate, followed by a further promotion to Associate Director.

I was approached by the Sanctuary Cove Project Manager, Neil Griggs, an ex-Canadian military officer to see if we would be interested in providing our services. I knew the site quite well from various boating trips. Whilst I thought the job to be a pipe dream (the area was best described as a mosquito infested swamp), I expressed our interest.

The developer was Mike Gore who I would describe as a likeable rogue. The job was probably beyond his financial capacity and experience, but he was very well connected politically. He managed to get the job to a stage where it could be sold, presumably at a good profit. Many of the ideas for Sanctuary Cove came from projects in Canada who Mike and his wife Jenny took a liking to. They liked Whistler ski resort for the way the town was laid out. They also liked Granville Island which is in Central Vancouver and is an old industrial area converted into a retail and tourist area. Two firms of Canadian architects who worked on the above projects were employed on Sanctuary Cove. A local Gold Coast firm was also employed.

The residential part of the site was planned to be a gated community, with secure entries and private roads. Being a private estate, the developer was responsible for providing all services which would normally be done by Councils or supply authorities. NDY were asked to design the electrical supply and communications services. In those days, the only communication services normally provided were basic telephone services care of Telstra. NDY designed a multifunctional system which provided security monitoring and an early version of what we now see on the internet as well as telephone.

Following the early planning the job was paused for several years. One basic problem was that the laws in Australia did not allow gated communities and private ownership of roads and services. It took several years for the enabling legislation to get through the Queensland Parliament. When it did get through, the pressure was on to progress the design.

The Architect was in Vancouver and the rest of the design team on the Gold Coast. In those days the technology which would enable working apart did not exist and the Architect was not able to move his staff immediately to the Gold Coast. So, the answer was for the Structural Engineer (John Stone of Burchill and Partners) and myself as Mechanical Engineer to go to Vancouver to coordinate with the architect. The build requiring our input was the Hyatt Regency Hotel (now the Intercontinental). Structure and air conditioning require the most coordination, with other services requiring less space.

We managed to pull together the planning and then John and I spent a few days in the Rockies and had a stopover in San Francisco on the way home.

During my time I was invited to join Rotary and did so. This started a long association which is still going after 40 years. Rotary has taught me leadership from a different perspective and contributed to my development in many areas.

Chapter 8 – NDY Queensland. 1977 to 1987

The NDY Willow Benders competed in an indoor cricket tournament with the other teams provided by engineering consultants, architects, and quantity surveyors. The first lesson learned was to bowl first if you win the toss. You can't drink when fielding but may succumb to a few ales when waiting to bat. On one occasion, my good friend Don Miller was batting under the influence and collided with a fieldsman and put his teeth through his lower lip. He finished his batting spell and the game ended. Don had a beer using a straw which he inserted through the split in his lip, and I then took him to the hospital for the required stitches.

We also competed in a touch football competition. I hadn't played Rugby League for quite a while and touch certainly tested the fitness level.

In 1985, my marriage with Margaret ended and I rented a unit on the Gold Coast. Belinda, Jodie and Danielle were with me every second weekend.

Later that year I met Deborah who I would later marry. Deborah had a twin sister Judith and another pair of twin sisters, Catherine and Margaret who were a couple of years older. There were also three brothers. At one stage the family had 6 children under school age. The girls are very close and God help any of the husbands who transgress in any way.

My father Jack died in May after a prolonged spell in Hospital.

In the early 80's I started working out at the gym and lost considerable weight. This was no doubt influenced by the impending marriage split up. I have maintained membership of gyms ever since, with the type of gym influenced by my health situation and age.

In 1987, I was given the opportunity to transfer to New Zealand where David Norman had identified some significant opportunities and wanted to me to establish and run the new office.

Deborah had been accepted for a role as Flight Attendant with Qantas International. By choosing the right flights or flying at staff rates she would be able to spend a lot of her time in Auckland. My daughters could spend school holidays with us.

Chapter 9. NDY New Zealand
1997 to 1990

Arriving in a new country and having to set up a new business would be a challenge at any time. In 1987, there was a major boom under way. New Zealand was in the early days of deregulation instigated by the labour government and Prime Minister David Lange. Office space was hard to get and very expensive. Telephones took several months to install and could not be applied for without a property being owned or leased.

We managed to pick up a project about the time I landed. It was a 30 storey Office Tower in Auckland. With no staff, no office, no home, and no phone it presented a real challenge.

A local Civil/Structural Engineer had some spare space which they allowed me to use. I also used (or more correctly, overused) their telephone. I looked to find a rental unit which was set up to suit a businessman and most importantly had a phone line. I was lucky enough to find a very nice unit in the beautiful suburb of Devonport.

Having no staff, I was reliant on work being done in Sydney. It was prior to the days of Computer Aided Drafting and drawings were produced by hand on transparent film. Whilst the drawings were sent by courier, that was not quick enough to keep up with the project. So, the drawings were printed in Sydney and the prints were sliced into A4 wide portions, the length of the drawing in height. I would arrive home in the evening to find a tangle of drawing strips and had to put together a "jigsaw" to work out what belonged where. Then sticky tape was used to put together a full drawing. Occasionally I would have a paper jam and had to work out what was missing and have them resent.

Gradually we recruited staff – some from other offices and others locally. I had learned from previous experience on the Gold Coast that the social situation in the office was fundamental to creating the right workplace. We were very social indeed.

Bob Meggitt was sent to Auckland from Brisbane where he had commenced as a graduate Electrical Engineer. Bob was 2IC to me and performed very well. It was difficult to recruit staff which reflected the overheated financial situation.

I joined a gym soon after arriving in Auckland, not wanting to allow my fitness to slip, and retained my membership throughout my stay.

Our project proceeded well. The developer required the building to be constructed using steel beams. The developer had a subsidiary company which specialised in steel fabrication. Steel construction had been avoided for many years in Australia and NZ because both countries had encountered major union problems and delays with steel buildings.

Chapter 9 – NDY New Zealand. 1997 to 1990

So, a new challenge for me. We worked closely with the Architect and Structural Engineer to come up with a solution which kept the ceiling space requirements to a reasonable level. Part of the solution was to provide oval penetrations through the steel beams. It was necessary to increase the beam depth by 80 mm which then allowed for 300 high oval penetrations in the beams for ductwork, cable trays and piping.

The project design was completed when the Developer had a significant change of staff. The new team decided they did not want the project to be constructed in steel and appointed a new design team to provide a more traditional NZ design. Whilst this was a shame, our fees were fully paid so financially the outcome was good.

The Auckland Savings Bank required a new headquarters and NDY was appointed for the building services. The job proceeded to schematic design and went to the ASB Board for approval on Tuesday, October 20, 1987. For those who remember that black Monday on the New York Stock Exchange was on the 19th, so we were very pessimistic on the chance of approval. However, the project was approved that day, and this was to provide us with a good workload in a very difficult period following the stock market crash.

Ross Legh was transferred from the NDY KL office. Ross is a very competent Mechanical Engineer and manager and his transfer to NZ was with a view to him taking over management of the NZ operation. There were plans for me to take on more senior roles within the company. At NDY's

Board Meeting of August 1987, I was appointed as a shareholder of the company. I was immediately appointed to the Executive group which consisted of a handful of senior partners. At that time discussion was under way regarding the possibility of me taking the role of Sydney Director which was held by Alan Disney who planned to retire in 1989.

NDY also was appointed for the Majestic Building in Wellington – another high-rise office tower. When the developer purchased the site, it was massive hole in the ground. One historic house was retained and it sat on a column of rock on the edge of the site. The building was operating at that time as a brothel. As you would no doubt understand, many site surveys were required.

We did a schematic design for a high rise office building in Queen St, Auckland. The project was unique in that the site was an extinct volcano. The volcano itself had a core of basalt in the shape the edge of the of an inverted cone. The building we were looking at would sit on the corner of the cone. The challenge for the team – how big a building could safely be supported on the site? It also became an exercise in reducing the weight of the structure which in turn would provide additional floor area.

During this time my relationship with Deborah flourished. NZ was not a highly sought after route for Qantas Flight Staff. There was also a route from Sydney to LA via Auckland which gave her two days in Auckland. Then she could work back to Sydney and return to Auckland under staff travel and, as her partner, I was entitled to staff rates. Given staff fares are "subject to load", I could not risk

Chapter 9 – NDY New Zealand. 1997 to 1990

travelling at peak times for fear of not being able to return home for my work. But we did take advantage of it many times for overseas trips.

We were a few years together without having lived together full time and decided to take a long trip to UK and Europe in 1988. A trial honeymoon. We had a great time and travel became very much part of our lives.

In August 1989 the NDY Directors and Managers Meeting was held on the Gold Coast. Deborah and I decided to get married their after the meetings so our families could attend. This occurred at the Sheraton Mirage, a project which I had been very involved with. Deborah was raised on the Gold Coast, so it was an ideal arrangement.

We bought a house together in Devonport. It was an Edwardian Villa which backed onto Mount Victoria, one of the many extinct volcanoes in Auckland. We renovated and extended the property and were very proud of what we achieved.

I joined the Rotary Club of Devonport which I enjoyed for the three years I was in Auckland. It was a very good club, and I enjoyed my time there. Unfortunately, my workload was such that I could not put as much time as I would have liked into the club. It provided another network of friends in Auckland.

Belinda, Jodie and Danielle flew over during the school breaks. One holiday was a trip on camper van around the South Island. Winter trips were often to Mt Ruapehu where we all went skiing. They really were fun times. When the girls weren't with me, I often went down with Ross and Margaret Legh for weekends. A 4:00 am start and we were on the way to Lake Taupo where we would have a picnic breakfast with Mt Ruapehu forming a background and the lake in the foreground. We would then drive onto the mountain in time for the opening of the ski lift. A full day skiing, a night in a lodge, then Sunday skiing before heading back to Auckland utterly exhausted.

Another highlight for Devonport was the ferry service from the city. It was an old steam ferry. the Kestrel. It was driven by a 12-cylinder steam engine which could be observed through windows from the deck. A steam engine can operate equally well in reverse, so that the vessel did not have to turn 180 degrees to moor. The was a wheelhouse at either end of the boat and the skipper went to the opposite end for the return trip. However, the most attractive part of the boat was the bar which featured a traditional jazz band. Many a Steinie was downed whilst the band played "Won't You Come Home Bill Bailey".

Our time in Auckland was coming to an end. We held a party on a Sunday afternoon. One of the staff was able to obtain a freshly killed pig. We cooked it on a gas BBQ, on a spit. It was wonderful meal and perhaps we had a slight access of incohol.

Chapter 10. NDY Sydney 1990 to 2007

Prior to transferring to Sydney, the firm sponsored me to undertake the Advanced Management Program at Mt Eliza in Melbourne. The college at Mt Eliza was previously the home of Sir Reginald Ansett of Ansett Airlines fame. I was sort of a mini-MBA aimed at people who were already in management positions but could benefit from the course. It was live in for 5 weeks and included lectures morning, afternoon and evening 7 days a week with one weekend off in the middle of the course. I learned a lot about understanding other people and about myself. One key thing I took away was that when issues were discussed, I should give weighting to the person who had the most knowledge in the subject. This may not be the person talking the most. This has served me well.

An interesting attendee at the course was a matron who had worked her way to a senior position in charge of a great number of nurses. She had spent her career in an era when doctors were predominately male, and nurses were female. She was a very highly intelligent person, and I enjoyed her company at meals, when she was very personable. She saw her role as protecting her nurses from the unreasonable requirements of doctors. The attendees at the Mt Eliza course were predominately male. When matters were discussed at meetings, she could become very aggressive for no apparent reason. I can remember one exercise where a team was to prioritise a number of steps to take to solve a problem. Each person did this alone, and then the team was asked to do it together. If the team got a score greater than that achieved by any individual, the team had a positive synergy. Early in the discussion, our matron debated a point with a male member of the team and ended up refusing to talk for the rest of the exercise. As it turned out, she had 100% on her own and the team got considerably less than that – our synergy sucked.

I arrived in Sydney in May 1990. The challenges before me were quite daunting. Firstly, the Auckland and Gold Coast Offices had about 20 staff. Sydney had 120 plus. The other factor was whether the senior staff would accept a new leader much younger than them.

Deborah and I were provided with accommodation and rented a unit in Blues Point Tower. This was paid for by the company as part of my relocation package. Blues Point is a small peninsular on the North Shore of the Harbour. This would be the first time that we had lived together on a permanent basis. It was within walking distance of North Sydney, Milsons Point and the ferry terminal which delivered us into Circular Quay and the city. Blues Point Tower was designed by one of Australia's greatest architects, Harry Seidler. NDY had worked closely with Harry for many years and there was little doubt that I would be working with Harry in the future. The building was the first of what was to be a series of high-rise structures to provide for increased population. However, a new council abandoned the development and Blues Point Tower stood alone, looking strangely out of place. The suburb was a quiet little backwater in the heart of Sydney. We thoroughly enjoyed our time there.

We were not able to sell our house in Auckland, so rented a house in Seaforth. In 1991, interest rates for mortgages dropped from 17% to 13% and we thought it was time to buy a property. Sydney prices are prone to rise rapidly, and we wanted to get our foot in the door. The market had lifted in Auckland, and we were able to sell our house, albeit at substantial loss. Shortly after this, NZ won the America's cup and the value of the property went through the roof.

We bought a house in Balgowlah Heights which was literally the worst house in a good street. We had very little money and did a lot of work ourselves. Income from my NDY shareholding was enough for us to employ contractors to do the work I was not capable of doing.

In 1999, we decided to sell the house and buy something better. We made a good profit on our investment. We identified a property in Clontarf which was built over 3 levels. There was a very nice pool and the third level at the rear of the property. It had magnificent views of the Harbour and Balmoral. We remodelled the property, and in particular extended the deck at the front of the house, which had the view of the Harbour.

NDY's offices were in St Leonards, a short drive or train trip from North Sydney. David Norman had put together team of investors to develop the building in the early

1970s. Partners in the venture included Leo Addicoat (A partner in Norman and Addicoat), Alan Disney, Bruce Sinclair and Jock Knight. Sinclair and Knight were the founding partners of Sinclair Knight, later renamed Sinclair Knight Merz and more recently merged with the Jacobs Engineering Group. At the time of construction in 1974, it was the tallest building between North Sydney and the Gold Coast, standing at 10 office floors plus a plant room at Level 11.

It had a unique structure and construction method. The lift core and columns were constructed to the full height of the building. Then the 11th floor structure was poured at ground level and hoisted into place using appropriately located jacks. The structure was lifted a little high to allow concrete pins to be inserted through holes left in the columns and lift core. The slab and beams were then lowered into their final location. Many years later I was on the phone to a colleague when I exclaimed "Shit, that was an earthquake." And it was a tremor which was felt in various locations in Sydney. The upthrust of the tremor caused the slab and beams to lift by a minor amount and fall back down, causing the notable shudder I so eloquently described. The tremor was generally not felt in other buildings which had a conventional structure.

David was the major shareholder in the building and managed the building in house. There was a fulltime building manager and various contractors for regular service and repairs. NDY was expanding, and an increasing amount of David's time was being spent interstate or overseas. He requested me keep an eye on things in his absence and signing cheques for service providers. I remember signing the last mortgage payment.

Sydney Office was the original NDY office and was very strongly moulded by David Norman who had built up a formidable team of Air Conditioning Engineers. Most of our research and development and associated technical guidance documentation originated in Sydney. This documentation provides guidance to our younger staff (and sometimes our more experienced staff) and was fundamental to maintaining NDY's position at the forefront of Air Conditioning Consulting Engineers.

As a young engineer, I had frequently referred to the R & D documentation prepared by these people and would also seek advice on issues I was not up to speed with. Assistance was always provided, and that attitude was a cornerstone on which David Norman established the practice. I started as a Junior Engineer and these guys helped me to develop my skills to a level where I was approaching their level of proficiency. And I was appointed to manage them — I felt quite inadequate in many ways, and it took some time for me to become confident in my own ability relative to the many mentors I had in the Sydney Office.

A key mentor on air conditioning design was Bill Drew who was the leading man in the area, and the best engineer I have ever worked with. Unfortunately, he did not come across confidently in meetings and much of his work was done behind the scenes. Prior to my arrival in Sydney, Bill had completed a degree in Computer Sciences at an age when most people were winding down. Bill was a shy but friendly character and I enjoyed my friendship with him. Even after his retirement, I was able to coax him back to assist me on a couple of major projects.

He wrote the NDY heat load program, which calculates the air flow and air temperatures required throughout an air conditioning system. This was an excellent program, being very user friendly. And Bill was there to resolve any bugs or issues which occurred. It served the company very well for many years and compared favourably with commercially available programs.

My predecessor was Alan Disney who had joined the business whilst still at university. David mentored him and at the time of formation of Norman Disney & Young, Alan was appointed as manager of the Sydney Office, with David being CEO with responsibilities for the overall organisation which by then included offices in Sydney, Melbourne, and Perth. Alan was very much a people person, quite an unusual but valuable trait for an engineer.

In the time leading up to my arrival in Sydney, the property market in Sydney had gone from boom to bust. There were six huge projects cancelled in Sydney on which NDY were employed. In 1989, we had employed a large number of staff in a very tight market. We still had an insufficient number of staff. Good staff were hard to find and quite a few of the recently employed staff were of questionable ability. Then the downturn hit. Alan confessed to me on arrival that a culling of staff was needed, but he could not undertake such an unpleasant task.

Chapter 10 – NDY Sydney 1990 to 2007

In the first few months I worked through a retrenchment program which occurred in two steps. Being the new guy on the block who was wielding the axe, I am sure my image with staff was very poor indeed. I kept the staff informed on our situation. Several senior members of staff approached with a suggestion that we go to reduced working hours. This had very wide support and was implemented for six months at which time we were able to return to full time employment.

Sydney Office made quite a reasonable profit in the early 90's despite this major downsizing, which was vital to the financial health of the wider organisation. I became accepted by the staff over time.

One issue which did cause consternation amongst staff early was my decision to ban smoking in the office. We had quite a few heavy smokers. My decision was in advance of the legislation which was introduced by Government. My thinking was
- NDY were a firm which understood the issues involved in smoking, including passive smoking.
- The best medical advice was (and still is) that there is no safe level of cigarette smoke.
- An employer could be open to claims from non-smokers should they suffer a medical problem attributable to cigarette smoke.

This occurred while retrenchments were happening. My thinking was that we best get all the bad news dealt with and then move on in a more positive atmosphere. That worked well.

Soon after arriving in Sydney, I was given my first problem job to sort out. NDY had designed the Air Conditioning as part of a refurbishment of the historic Katoomba Court House. We had not been involved in the construction phase, that role being handled by the responsible government authority. When the system was put into operation it was unable to cope with the heating required in winter. Katoomba is in the Blue Mountains west of Sydney and has cool winters with snow falling several times a year.

The people looking after the project determined that the problem was the way the air condition was designed. The court rooms were about 4 m high, and air was supplied at high level and return air was also taken from high level. Hot air rises and the theory was that the warm air was suspended at high level and the room remained cold. The government modified the building to provide for low level return. The modifications were quite expensive and disruptive but failed to fix the heating problem. They advised NDY of the issue and indicated we may be held responsible.

No one from NDY had inspected the site during or after the construction. The problem as described above was a plausible reason for the heating problem. However, it was strange that the low-level return air did not work. I arranged to visit the site with a senior guy from the government. When we arrived at the courthouse, there was snow on the ground and temperature were below freezing. Ideal conditions for investigating a heating problem.

When I walked into the courthouse, I could feel a chill in my feet which permeated through the soles of my shoes. A few quick measurements showed the air at high level was not warm and the supply air was cool – about 12 ^{0} C whereas it should be about 30 ^{0} C. This indicated a problem with the plant and an inspection showed that the contractor had failed to install control dampers for the outside air. The system was operating on a much higher outside air quantity than it was designed for. This took us about 30 mins. We went to the newsagent and purchased some cardboard and adhesive tape, returned to site, and sealed up most of the outside air grille. Then off to the historic Parthenon Milk bar in Katoomba for a coffee. We returned to site to find staff complaining the Air Conditioning was too hot - a sure sign we were on the right path, and we returned to Sydney after making a couple of control adjustments..

My colleague in the government was during this friendly and competent. He rang me a few weeks later to advise the contractor had permanently fixed the defects and all was well. He enquired whether NDY was prepared to assist with the costs of the (unnecessary) modifications made to the building and I advised him we weren't. I am sure that come as no surprise.

As things improved, the office won many projects, and each had a senior person responsible for the management of the job, As the Director, I also managed several projects at any one time. I tended to take on complex projects or projects where the client relationships were important.

This put me in a position to work on a never-ending stream of challenging jobs with interesting project teams which might involve Architects, Project Managers, Structural Engineers, Quantity Surveyors, and client representatives. Sometimes NDY were appointed for all Building Services in which case I would coordinate the work of all our specialised disciplines. In the early days of my time in Sydney we were very strong in Air Conditioning with the electrical side of the business being relatively small. So sometimes our opposition firms were employed on the project as well.

I developed a wide range of contacts throughout the industry and developed many friendships.

One of the first major projects I worked on was Angel Place which is in a small laneway not far from St Martin's Place in the heart of Sydney. The project was a 40 floor office tower with an adjacent recital hall. The recital hall was paid for by the developer (AMP Society) and gifted to the council, this being in exchange for relaxation of council requirements on the office tower.

Richard Pickering was an English Mechanical Engineer who was relatively inexperienced when I arrived in Sydney but showed great promise. He was a very good designer and related well to people. He did the majority of the work, with me attending higher level meetings and reviewing the design as it progressed.

Whilst the office tower represented most of the work, the interesting and challenging bit was the recital hall. There are many such facilities in Europe and elsewhere. Some of them were built hundreds of years ago. The most fundamental issue is to be able to provide an excellent acoustic environment. Until the early 20th century, there was no electronic sound amplification and the sound needed to be heard at high quality by a large audience. One principal was that the hall dimension must approximate the proportions of a shoebox.

The role of the Acoustical Engineer was paramount. NDY were yet to establish an acoustical group and so we were working with an opposition firm who did an excellent job. Our hall was to have an audience capacity of 1250. The typical performance would be a small chamber music group which would not have sound reinforcement. The hall was to be flexible enough to cater for many activities including such diverse activities as a symphony orchestra or a company AGM.

The site was very close to the Martin Place underground station, which was built many years ago and, in those days, scant regard was paid to the vibration caused by trains. Structural borne is very difficult to predict and if it was to be transmitted to the recital hall structure, the problems would be immense. The acoustic engineers provided rubber isolation pads on which the whole recital hall was supported. These are similar to car engine mounts but much larger.

The noise level of operating equipment was set at a figure below the threshold of hearing. This is a particular challenge for us as the air conditioning designers. The level of noise created by air flowing through supply grilles would exceed the noise level required, even at the lowest velocity conceivable. We used a computer program (computational fluid dynamics) to assist us in coming up with a solution.

We supplied the air at high level via a low velocity duct, the air being discharged through an opening (no grille). The temperature of the supply needed to be higher than normal air conditioning systems. If the air was too cool, it would drop rapidly down and cause discomfort. Our initial computer runs showed that the air was unstable, and this was addressed by providing return air outlets below the floor into the void created by the tiered seating. The balconies required return air as well. When installed the system operated as predicted by the computer study.

The opening act was David Helfgott, who was a brilliant musician despite suffering from enormous mental issues. He was the subject of the movie Shine in which Geoffrey Rush played David. I was with a few of the design team on the day prior to opening and we found ourselves next to David and his wife and carer Gillian. When they found out we were responsible for the design, they were both in tears and excited about performing in this new world class venue. They thanked us for creating such a wonderful hall. David was touching all of us as he spoke, and it reinforced what a magnificent job Geoffrey Rush did in the movie. Only a brief moment, but one I shall cherish forever.

On opening night Deborah and I were guests and David Helfgott was wonderful, but I had great difficulty enjoying the performance. Every now and then a fan would start up and it would sound like a trolley bus. Then it would

Chapter 10 – NDY Sydney 1990 to 2007

stop with a similar noise. I knew exactly which item of equipment it was coming from. The following day the Sydney Morning Herald was quite critical of the facility.

The next day, I consulted Dick Winchcombe, who was another a mentor of mine in the Sydney Office and specialised in the construction phase of projects. Dick had an incredible knowledge of the practical issues in air conditioning. He had experienced a similar problem with the air cooled condenser fans which were made in China. The fans were low speed (570 rpm). The lower the speed, the more difficult it is to manufacture the motors and the motor will hum if the windings are poor, which they were. We worked out a solution with the air conditioning contractor who obtained higher speed (900 rpm) motors and installed them within a week. This was satisfactory in the interim until speed controllers could be provided to reduce the fan speed to 570 rpm.

A few months later and our AMP client invited Deborah and I to a function in one of the smaller rooms in the complex. We were entertained by Simon Tedeschi, a young pianist at that time. There were only a dozen or so people attending and to experience such a wonderfully talented performer so close up was amazing. Simon had actually played the piano in the movie Shine. All you can see of him in the movie is his hands at the keyboard.

I was very hands on in the SBS radio and tv studios at Artarmon. Prior to this SBS had their studios in an old and very basic office building in Milson's Point. The only area they transmitted from was a desk behind which the newsreaders sat. Above them was a host of equipment hidden by a ceiling dropped so low that the newsreaders could not stand upright.

They purchased the old John Sands warehouse and manufacturing facility. The job had a tight budget and was awarded to Baulderstone on a Design and Construct basis. We were part of Baulderstone's team. SBS's wish was list quite extravagant despite the low budget. It showed every sign of being a difficult job which was why I chose to act as the project coordinator for NDY.

A key debate was the number and size of TV studios and the degree of sound isolation required. SBS wanted 2 studios - one with an audience capacity of 100 and the other 400. I can recall a meeting where I made the statement "You don't have a viewing audience of 400". I have a rather cynical sense of humour and fortunately it was accepted as a joke.

Regarding noise, the site was close to Royal North Shore Hospital, and TV Channels 7, 9 and 10. All of these used helicopters on a regular basis. If the studios were to achieve the low background noise levels needed for TV production, the cost of acoustic treatment would be prohibitive. If the TV Studios were live to air, the treatment would be necessary. If the show was being recorded, it would be possible to retake any segment spoiled by helicopter noise. SBS had difficulty making the necessary compromises to keep the job within budget.

Eventually, Brian Johns, MD of SBS and later MD of the ABC, called a meeting and went through the issues which needed to be addressed. He was a very impressive character and agreed where compromises were needed to enable the budget to be met. Given the tightness of the budget and the relatively low probability a helicopter would pass close by during filming, the decision was made not to provide the acoustic treatment required to silence helicopter noise.

Baulderstone performed well and the result was a very good project.

As it turned out, I never got to work on a major project with Harry Seidler which was unfortunate. I did work on a few smaller projects and proposals with him. His offices and his apartment were in Milsons Point and to the west overlooked the Luna Park. When Luna Park applied for permission to build their roller coaster, Harry was a prominent objector but was not able to stop it being build. On one occasion, Harry invited me into the apartment, and I accepted the invitation eagerly. Harry's architectural style was minimalist, and his lounge was exactly as it would have been presented for a photo shoot. Tiled floors and exposed beams, a lounge suite, a glass table and a single vase and that was it.

The Sydney Olympic Aquatic Centre was awarded to Lend Lease. NDY has had a very close relationship with Lend Lease, both firms being founded at a similar time in Sydney. Lend Lease engaged NDY for Mechanical Services. This project was commenced well before the vote for the successful City for the year 2000 Olympics, as a tangible demonstration of Sydney's commitment to the event.

The Public Works Department had a close overview of the project and the set up was very political. Given the importance of the project, I took up the role of Project Director and once again Richard Pickering handled the air conditioning design.

Architects for the project were Cox, Richardson and Associates, with John Richardson being the senior contact. They have a strong reputation for "Large Span" projects such as entertainment centres, art galleries and sporting stadiums. I enjoyed a good relationship with the Cox guys.

Lend Lease employed Bob Johnstone, a young graduate electrical engineer from Townsville to act as the services coordinator for the project. He did an outstanding job despite his lack of experience. Within a few years, Lend Lease took over the Bovis group. The purchase included a substantial number of properties in USA which were of concern. Bob was given the task of sorting out the problems, which included deciding which projects to retain and which should be sold. A few more years and he was appointed as the CEO of the Lend Lease Group worldwide, operating from London. He left Lend Lease after this role but was greatly admired in the organisation.

Aquatic centres usually have hot and humid spectator areas. The Aquatic Centre brief required air conditioning of the spectator areas which had never been done in any aquatic centre in the world. The key problem was that the pool water temperature is required to be 27 deg C. For the comfort of the swimmers, the pool surround was required to be approximately 29 deg C. The spectator area was to be approximately 23 deg C.

Cold air falls and since the spectator area is a tiered space above the pool, the air would tend to fall to the pool surrounds, and the temperature would be too low for the comfort of the swimmers. We used computer modelling (computational fluid dynamics) to come up with a solution. It used a warm air flow at the bottom of the spectator area to hold up the cooler air in the spectator area to prevent it falling onto the pool surrounds. The actual installation went as predicted by the modelling.

We were also required to provide heating for the pool water. Various heating methods were considered including gas, solar and heat reclaim. The centre was designed to be a public pool and fitness centre and was expected to be used for long hours. The best alternative was to use the waste heat from an air conditioning chiller which effectively provides free heating. The centre had more patronage by the public than expected, so the heating performance exceeded expectations.

Whilst NDY did not have a role in the main stadium, I was keen to attend the opening event which was the Bee Gees one night only concert. We invited several clients, and a great evening was had by all. One irritation was that the image on the Video Screens was out of synch with the sound. The press had a great time criticising the stadium facilities, but the fact is that all of the video and sound gear was brought in on a 747 by the Bee Gees and it was their production people who got it wrong.

The Superdome was the major indoor venue for the Olympics having a seating capacity of 15,000 which catered for such sports as basketball and gymnastics. The tender was let on a build own operate basis and was won by Abigroup. NDY were the services consultants. Once again Cox Richardson and Partners were the architects.

We designed a displacement air conditioning system. Basically, this system provides cool air at say 20 deg C at low level. The heat of the bodies induces an upward flow of air which is returned to the system at high level. This system has become popular in entertainment centres as it is highly energy efficient. Normally the system used seats which integrated the supply air. However, the cost of these seats was very high. So, our design used supply air grilles located in the upstands of the terraced seating.

The design was computer modelled (computational fluid dynamics). There was some concern that the provision of cool air might cause discomfort and it was decided to build a full scale model of a section of seating, complete with air conditioning. The set up was tested by many of the design team and it was agreed to be satisfactory, and the system design was finalised.

I was fortunate to be invited to Abigroup's corporate box for the opening performance by Pavarotti. Another treasured memory for the very harmonious relationships between NDY, Abigroup, Cox Richardson and Partners and the entire design team. Not all projects work like that.

Chapter 10 – NDY Sydney 1990 to 2007

Given our participation in the design and construction of games facilities, we thought it appropriate to do some client entertainment at games events. We purchased four packages which gave us considerable access to leading events. I was fortunate enough to attend the opening ceremony - another lifelong memory created. I also went to the athletics one evening where the highlight for me was the finish of the women's marathon. This was at the time Australia had a peacekeeping force in East Timor, and a young Timorese lady was one of the stragglers in the event. On entering the stadium, she sunk to the ground and bowed to the Aussie spectators. One of the officials advised her that she had to complete a lap which she did to a rousing cheer.

I thought I had picked a great night for the swimming with Ian Thorpe and Madam Butterfly Susie O'Neill red hot favourites to win gold in the Aquatic Centre which I had worked on. Unfortunately, both were relegated to second place, and consequently I have never seen the Aussies win a gold medal.

Deborah is not a sports fan, but she does enjoy the gymnastics, and was seconded to host some female clients to the Superdome, the other project I had been heavily involved in.

The feel we experienced in Sydney during the games was amazing. I can recall catching the ferry at Manly destined for Circular Quay. The sailing was taking place at the time, and the ferry had to take a circuitous route at low speed. The trip took 90 mins instead of 20. We had on board a group of Brazilian buskers who decided to entertain us.

The passengers spontaneously started singing and it all became a bit of a party.

As this was all happening, the company was preparing for the retirement of David Norman. David had restructured the company in anticipation of the retirement of the first generation of shareholders. He set up a partnership agreement which was very attractive to incoming shareholders. I benefitted from that as an incoming shareholder and passed on a similar benefit to younger shareholders as I approached retirement.

Ian Hopkins was the heir apparent. Ian had started as a graduate in the Sydney Office in the early 1970's. After a couple of years, he resigned and took up a role with an air conditioning contractor in Adelaide, quickly rising to state manager despite his young age.

A few years later, NDY had a parting of the ways with founding director Peter Young who was responsible for the Melbourne office. David Norman managed to convince Ian to take up the role as manager of Melbourne. Ian was responsible for major growth of the office from about 20 to 150 in a very short time frame. He was the obvious candidate to replace David.

David was both the CEO and the Managing Director of the company. He relinquished the role of MD to Ian. At that time, I started to work more closely with Ian and we developed a very good working relationship, as well as a close personal relationship which remains in place despite us having retired long ago.

David remained CEO until 1994 when he retired. Ian became CEO and retained the role of MD, with planning put in place to groom another MD. I was appointed as Deputy CEO.

Upon David's retirement I somewhat reluctantly moved into his office - I did not feel worthy of that. But we did not want to refurbish at the time, and this was the only logical solution.

In addition to my responsibilities in the Sydney Office, I was taking more responsibility at corporate level. I had been appointed to the board in 1997 whilst I was still in New Zealand. I was the youngest director and found myself responsible for IT. My skills in the area were not great but probably the best of the directors of the time. It was really a matter of listening to our IT people, developing an understanding of the issues, and making recommendations. The most significant initiative was a decision to change from Hewlett Packard Computer Aided Drafting system to AutoCAD. Our HP equipment was superior to AutoCAD at the time, but we foresaw that AutoCAD was rapidly expanding and the third-party software companies were producing software tailored to AutoCAD. This included engineering software which is vital to the firm's ability to be at the leading edge.

I found IT work somewhat frustrating. Every time a system was developed, it always seemed to take considerably longer that programmed. This seems to be endemic in the whole IT area and certainly not confined to NDY – Microsoft and Apple seem to have similar issues. And once software is issued, then come the inevitable upgrades and bug fixes. I always was encouraged when the IT guys said they were 95% complete because you knew you were halfway there. But that reflects my impatience and I understand just how difficult IT processes can be and the guys did very well for NDY.

Fortunately, as engineers younger than myself were appointed to senior level, I was able to hand over the IT responsibility to people far more knowledgeable in that area than I.

Another task I was given in the early 90's was to establish a Quality Assurance System. Clients were increasingly requiring their service providers to have a QA System in place. The documentation of the system was a massive task which took me 2 years of work which was fitted in between my responsibilities on projects and management tasks. I didn't really enjoy the task and was driven by a sense of duty to get the task completed. Then there was training for our Sydney staff, implementing the system, and obtaining third party accreditation. All our offices required accreditation and I provided a support role in the process.

Our office accommodation in St Leonards was becoming dated. Clearly, we needed to provide better facilities for our staff. Given David Norman was the major shareholder in the building we occupied, it was a very touchy matter to consider leaving the premises. However, despite the enormous respect I have for David, my position required me to do what was best for NDY and I made the decision to rent premises in North Sydney. The move was very

Chapter 10 – NDY Sydney 1990 to 2007

popular with staff and the firm remains a tenant in the same building.

The electrical division in the office was under strength when I arrived and remained so for the first few years of my directorship. This changed when we were able to obtain the services of Tony Lukic. Tony was recruited in Melbourne as part of our graduate program and progressed rapidly. He had a particular interest in high tech facilities such as data centres.

NDY also had considerable experience in data centres due to our close association with the Optus roll out. We were part of the Leighton team which supported the Optus bid to be the second communications carrier in Australia. Included in the Optus team were British Telecom and Bell South from America. We had expected those parties to be knowledgeable in providing new data facilities. However, they had only done upgrades and refurbishments in recent times and we were left to work out the best way to provide the necessary data centres built from scratch and designed to handle only the latest equipment. This we did and we gained considerable knowledge in the area which put us at the leading edge in the world and would prove to be a vital component of our international expansion.

Tony managed to get us involved with Fox and we designed the services for their production facilities for cable TV.

Tony forged a close relationship with WorldCom, and we completed several data centres for them in the late 1990's, prior to their fall from grace. He was responsible for training recent graduates and our electrical team in Sydney grew in strength and ability.

Our key contact from WorldCom left the company and joined a start up company and was responsible for a roll out of data centres in the UK and Europe. He offered NDY the projects on the basis that we set up in the UK. This was a huge opportunity and so NDY expanded to London.

Tony went to London to set up the office in 1999. A few Australian staff went as well, including Richard Pickering, a very good Mechanical Engineer from the Sydney Office and staff were also recruited locally. In August Tony took a break and I spent 5 weeks in London to keep things moving. During that time, we recruited several staff and secured office apace and designed the fit out. The office was a refurbished older building close to the Old St tube station. Tony had employed Jean Lewis as a PA and she started while I was in London. In later years she transferred to Melbourne, and she is now PA to Sam Aloi, Australian Regional Manager. She has been appointed an Associate, a rare achievement for a non-technical employee. Jean has been very helpful to me over the years.

We were also employed for a refurbishment of Shellmex House, a 50,000 sq m art deco office building adjacent the Embankment Tube Station and the Savoy Hotel. It is a prominent landmark building on the North Bank of the Thames.

The Air Conditioning System required replacement and the building was built in 1930, well before air conditioning was invented. The building was not therefore designed to

Chapter 10 – NDY Sydney 1990 to 2007

have air conditioning and in particular lacked ceiling space. The best solution seemed to be chilled beams which had become popular in the UK. NDY had no experience in this technology. Our observations indicated that there were some installations which worked well and others not so well. Richard and I looked at the systems and visited test facilities and existing systems where we could physically experience the operation of the system. Based on our investigations, we decided a chilled beam solution should be implemented. The project went ahead on this basis and the system worked well. Based on the knowledge gained I wrote a design guide. NDY used chilled beams where appropriate from that time. I have used the system on other jobs and other engineers have adopted it for projects. We used it for our own premises in Melbourne and it served as a working example of the technology.

Tony Lukic remained in London and identified local Engineers who could manage the office. He returned to his hometown, Melbourne. At this time Ian Hopkins was both CEO and MD, and Tony was being groomed for the Managing Director role. It came as a surprise when Tony resigned from the firm.

Our Melbourne director Stuart Fowler took on the role an MD which he still retains. Stuart is a clear thinker and has performed well in the role. Sam Aloi was appointed the Australian Regional Manager.

During my time in Sydney, I instigated a client entertainment event whereby we hired a boat for the start of the Sydney to Hobart yacht race. We catered for 150 people and NDY became closely identified with the event which we carried out for more than 25 years. A lot of close friendships and client relationships were enhanced on the basis of the race start cruise.

In the year 1997, an incident occurred in a Data Centre we were consultants for. The cost of repair was assessed at $29 million. Whilst it seemed clear that a subcontractor I shall call ABC was responsible, that company refused to offer any payment and the matter went to court in 2003. There were 5 defendants including NDY. Construction litigations are usually complex and involve many parties and this one was no different. The week after the case started, I was driving to work when I heard on the news that HIH had gone into liquidation. Our insurers were a subsidiary of HIH, and this meant that we were left uninsured and would have to fund the legal fees as well as any costs for which we were found liable. We would also have to manage the conduct of the court case on a day-to-day basis, and that role fell upon me. When witnesses gave evidence which was relevant to NDY, I received a transcript in the late afternoon and needed to provide comments and suggestions to our legal counsel early the next morning.

The case took 6 months, so we had to pay the costs of our solicitors and legal counsel. In addition we were at risk if the judgement went against us. If we were assessed to be 20% responsible, the firm would have been insolvent. Our belief was that we had nil liability. Our auditors would not sign off on our accounts without us making a provision for a contingent liability. This was a potential problem as sometimes prospective clients ask to see the accounts. We were most concerned that the doubt on our situation would become known in the industry and result in us not being considered for some projects. Fortunately, this did not occur.

The plaintiff's case is run first, and the usual approach is that all defendants are united in discrediting the plaintiff's case. Our legal advice was that ABC were putting forward silly arguments and had gotten offside with the judge. Our tactic became to isolate ourselves from the ABC defence.

One amusing incident occurred when the judge asked whether a certain witness for ABC would be appearing. ABC's counsel advised that they had been unable to contact the witness and he would not be appearing. After the next recess the counsel for Optus requested permission to address the court. Basically, he said "Mi lord, by way of assisting my learned friend, I managed to find the witness' phone number in the phone book and have rung him during the recess. He says he is quite willing to give evidence." Of course, the purpose of this was to imply that ABC's counsel had mislead the judge. In such a circumstance the judge would be entitled to conclude the evidence of the witness would not have reflected favourably on ABC. And presumably the Judge's view of the ABC defence team was further tarnished.

Two of our staff were witnesses and, in his judgment, the Judge was very complimentary to them, praising their honesty and openness. I was programmed to give evidence as well, but our legal advisers thought we had won the case by that stage, and it was best not to call up any more witnesses who might make an error under cross examination. I was particularly proud of our witnesses and the professionalism and judgement they showed under extreme pressure.

The judgement was handed down several months later and NDY were exonerated. ABC were found responsible for the great majority of the costs, which had grown to $50 m by the time all the legal costs, we were able to claim back all our costs of the legal case.

I had acquired a good legal understanding because of this case. Until this time, the placing of professional indemnity insurance and the management of claims had been treated by the firm as an administrative issue. It was agreed that I would take the responsibility for legal and risk issues. Over time we employed two solicitors to assist in managing these matters.

When HIH went into receivership, government was talking about assisting victims of the collapse. I thought it best to make representation to my local member, Tony Abbott who was then Health Minister in the Howard government. The government did not end up providing any assistance to companies in our situation. During the process I got to know Tony quite well and joined the Liberal Party. I would attend his monthly breakfasts which involved a guest speaker who was always interesting and not necessarily a supporter of Tony. I would normally be asked to sit at the head table so got to chat with some very influential people. On one occasion, there was a Muslim lady who spoke on the issues facing Muslims in

Chapter 10 – NDY Sydney 1990 to 2007

Australia. I invited fellow NDY Director Ashak Nathwani who was of Indian descent but born, raised and educated in Uganda. He fled to Australia during the Idi Amin era, ended up with NDY and worked his way to a directorship. He became prominent in the Indian expat community and the Muslim community. Out guest speaker spoke and question time began. I was sitting next to Bronwyn Bishop who was muttering derogatory comments throughout the presentation. Ashak answered some of the questions at the invitation of our guest speaker. Bronwyn gave the vote of thanks which turned into a criticism. I thought it showed her as being very bigoted and I was embarrassed for our Muslim guests.

I had continued my association with Rotary by joining the Rotary Club of Balgowlah. I acted I almost all board positions at various times, including President in 2005/06. 1999 was the year of the republican referendum. I thought it would be a good idea to have a debate between senior monarchists and republicans as a fundraiser for the club. I suggested the matter to Tony who was the leader on the Monarchists in Australia and advised that John Howard had banned parliamentarians from commenting on the referendum. Some months later Tony rang me and advised that John Howard had decided to allow the Liberal parliamentarians to speak their mind. I immediately rang the Republican movement chairman who accepted the idea and asked if I had a preference for speakers. I suggested Tom Keneally, a prominent author of Irish decent and a staunch republican. He was a passionate supporter on the Manly Sea Eagles and a popular figure in the Manly area.

Each side of the debate added another speaker, and the Rotary Club nominated a high school student for each side. On the night, Tony asked the high school student to anchor the debate. Normally the anchor would be the best debater – Tony generously wanted to give the student the best experience possible. I think this probably resulted in the Republicans winning the debate in the minds of most of the audience. I was probably biased in that I am a republican supporter, a fact that I did not share with Tony.

On the day of the debate, I was contacted by a reporter for the Daily Mirror from London. It was held on the Saturday prior to the vote, and he had just flown in to cover the referendum. He searched the web to see what relevant events were being held and found our function and requested a ticket to the event. The coverage in the Daily Mirror was a two-page article and included reference to our Rotary Club and our president at the time, Jack Kellahan.

Tony and his wife and Deborah and I also shared an interest in the Spilstead Centre. Spilstead is a facility which assists abused and neglected children and is located in the grounds of Dalwood House in Seaforth. Tony would visit our Rotary club from time to time and would attend functions for Spilstead.

Spilstead operates similar to a pre-school, with specialist input into the development of the kids who attend. They have a high number of volunteers, and the children are given far more adult attention than a normal pre-school. Children who are in this situation will benefit greatly if the

Chapter 10 – NDY Sydney 1990 to 2007

intervention is at an early age. It gets much harder if the child does not receive sufficient support when young.

In 2003, I decided to see what I could do to support Spilstead. I asked the person in charge, Kerry Gwynn how I could help. Her answer was "Raise funds to employ a part time speech therapist". That seemed a bit more than I contemplated and I asked "How much will that cost". The answer was "$45,000". That was considerably more than I had in mind but I answered "OK". All the children who attend the school have speech difficulties – some relatively mild, others serious. I discussed this with the Rotary Club, and they agreed to take on the project which was called "Child's Play".

Various functions were held, and supporters contributed. Brian Offner was a Rotarian who I introduced to Rotary. I had also employed him at NDY as the Sydney accounts manager. His daughter Renee was a stunning young lady who had entered the Miss Australia Charity Queen contest. She was a cheer leader for the Manly Sea Eagles, and they supported her in the contest. She raised over $23,000 for Spilstead Centre and won the Charity Queen contest. As a side note, Brian took over the role in the Sydney office left vacant when Kristina Mertens was transferred to Head Office. Tragically, shortly after Kristian died due to a fall, Brian also had a fall whilst doing some landscaping for Renee, broke his neck and died.

We raised the $45,000 within a few months. Kerry then announced that they needed a Child Psychologist and so the fund raising continued. The Rotary Club helped commence a jumble sale which is held about 6 times a year. The cost of the specialised staff is as at 2022 $175,000 annually. Whilst these services are available from the government, it is on a very limited basis. Added to that there is a high no show rate from Spilstead's parents. They are more likely to attend appointments in Spilstead in a safe and known environment.

Tony Abbott for many years used to organise a pollie's bike ride where politicians from all parties would participate and raise funds. One year a donation of $20,000 was made to the Child's Play project. He is a much criticised figure in our politics. But I won't make a comment on that aspect. I found him to be very supportive of community organisations and am thankful for the effort made to support the charities I was involved in.

There is an annual Rock Night which not only is a fund raiser, but a great night out for Spilstead staff and volunteers.

I enjoyed continued good health for the early part of my role as Sydney Director and at one stage had not taken a day's sick leave in over 20 years. However, in the early 2000's I started having difficulty sleeping and suffering from chronic tiredness. I now believe this was an early symptom of Cushing's disease. Cushing's causes high cortisol levels, and cortisol (the stress hormone) controls the circadian rhythm. We should have low cortisol as we approach our sleep time, and the peak level of cortisol as we wake up. My cortisol levels were probably high 24 hrs per day, dramatically affecting my sleep.

I thought the chronic tiredness might be a sign of stress. I had been operating at high level for over 30 years. Whilst I did not feel as though stress was getting to me, chronic tiredness was getting me down to the extent that I advised the board that I would be looking to step down as a shareholder in 2009 at the very young age of 56.

I thoroughly enjoyed my job and drove myself to continuing to perform at a high level despite the sleep issues.

One aspect of my role which I thoroughly enjoyed was the recruitment and training of graduate engineers. It was a core value of NDY that we should give opportunities to young people. I had benefited from this policy and wanted to employ young people with a view to them having similar opportunities. Around the end of each year, we would attend various universities (Sydney, NSW, UTS and Wollongong) and do a presentation aimed to attract graduates to apply for positions. We went to considerable lengths to attract the best possible candidates which provided talented people to fill key roles in relatively short time.

Sydney Office would employ about 4 each year, depending on our circumstances. The candidates would be interviewed and short listed by Kevin Vidler, a retired director and close friend. Then I would interview the candidates and decide who to employ. I can recall one year I thought one of the candidates who was not short listed looked to be worthy of consideration and I added her to the short list. I interviewed Corrina Grace and thought she was outstanding.

Corrina was employed as a Mechanical Engineer. Within a year she was taking on some very complex projects and dealing with some very difficult clients. One of the difficult clients was Macquarie Bank. They were so impressed with her that they offered her a job which she accepted. She did not stay long there either. She had a visit to Guatemala and found some work in a bar. She got involved with the local, mainly indigenous, people and began to see how their lives could be improved by training the younger people in leadership skills and alternative sustainable methods of farming. She was cofounder of SERES, a charitable organisation which has implemented her ideas.

She maintained some contact with people at NDY and the NDY Charitable Trust started to support SERES financially. I was the founder of the Charitable Trust and Chairman for the first few years. I have continued my relationship with the Trust which sometimes supports Rotary Projects which I think may suit NDY's criteria.

The SERES property is very close to Volcan De Fuego which had a major eruption in 2018. Many lives were lost, and properties destroyed due to lava flows. SERES were very involved it assisting the victims of the disaster.

I was in contact with Corrina to see what assistance Rotary could provide. It was decided that the SERES land would be used to grow crops which could assist the disaster victims. It was also to be used as a training facility for the local people to be trained in sustainable farming techniques and alternative crops. Guatemala has a climate which has wet and dry seasons. During the dry season the lack of water is a major problem. There was also a problem with the surface water which had been badly polluted for many years, a situation which was made worse by volcanic ash and lava. A water well and irrigation system was needed.

I was able to obtain donations from my Rotary club, the Rotary Club of Broadwater Southport and several of the Rotary clubs and individual Rotarians. There was also a donation from Jim Sheldon from Denver Colorado who is a long-term supporter of SERES. I managed to obtain District Grants and a Global Grant. We worked in association with the Rotary Club of Escuintla in Guatemala who oversaw the project on a day to day basis.

I have never worked on a water well before but am familiar with all the components which make up the installation. Good for an old dog to learn new tricks.

Alan Edler was employed as a graduate mechanical engineer. He immediately stood out as a very promising young man. We were appointed for the refurbishment of a major office building in the Sydney CBD, and I decided I would take on the project with Alan doing the design so I could help him through the learning curve to reach the level required of an experienced engineer. I expected that I would need to keep closely involved. He was always one step ahead of me and had an instinct of how to go about the design process.

Alan was fast tracked through the organisation and is now one of the Senior Directors of the company.

Peter Koulos was employed as a graduate electrical engineer. He quickly developed his skills. He also became heavily involved in our QA system. He became a key member of the Sydney management team, then transferred to London before taking up a role as the senior engineer in the Dubai office where he once again reported to me. In recent years he has taken up employment with an opposition company.

We employed Sean Treweek as a mechanical graduate who worked in our energy and plant management (EPM) group which looks after existing installations. This is a difficult assignment for a young engineer, but Sean excelled. Unfortunately, he left the company. I did meet with him to discuss the possibility him coming back to NDY. He was open to the possibility but wanted to stay where he was for the foreseeable future. He subsequently has taken up a Directorship with NDY.

The Mechanical Engineers who made the Sydney office a centre of excellence were reaching retirement age, and I approached Alan Irwin who had an excellent reputation. He had the advantage of having skills in the industrial engineering as well as air conditioning. He was not happy with his current employer, and I managed to recruit him. Alan was an great mentor for the young staff and sometimes for me. He also had experience in industrial projects, including the services required in traffic tunnels. His experience included the Sydney Harbour tunnel, which was completed about the time he joined NDY. In the future his expertise would be instrumental in our diversification into tunnel services.

Chapter 10 – NDY Sydney 1990 to 2007

The office required a bookkeeper to handle the financial management of our projects, plus handle purchase items, invoices and debtors. I employed Kristian Mertens, a young guy who was studying part time towards and accounting degree. Within a few years Kristian had outgrown the role and we gave him a role in head office assisting the Chief Financial Officer. On the CFO's retirement Kristian, who by then had completed his study and was a Certified Professional Accountant, was appointed to the role.

Kristian would often seek my counsel. NDY wanted to work out ways of providing benefits to staff which would be of value and assist in staff retention. An example which I am proud of was the implementation of an income replacement policy which paid out salaries during prolonged sickness. As it turned out I was a beneficiary of this initiative when I was off work for several months due to my Cushing's disease. Tragically Kristian had a fall which caused major brain damage and died several months later at the age of 43 without ever regaining consciousness. At least his partner and children were well taken care of financially. Kristian was borne on 8th of March 1974 which is the same day as my daughter Belinda. On that day I always recall him with fondness.

The other innovation we worked closely on together was the NDY Charitable Trust. The NDY directors had always been generous in their donations, but the approach was haphazard and our employees had limited input. The trust is run by a committee of staff representatives from each office. Each office has a committee to generate the support in the office and handle funding of local charities. The company donates a generous amount each year. About one third of this is set aside for agreed work in third world countries. The rest is distributed out to each office for them to support local charities. In addition, the offices and the Trust committee conduct various fund-raising events to increase the amount which can be donated. I was the Chairman on the Trust initially until my retirement when the role was handed over to Sam Aloi, the Australian Regional Manager. Sam is a wonderful people person and I think does a far better job that I in his role with the trust. I set up the guidelines for donations and these were driven by the principals I had learned in many years of Rotary. When I see a project which meets the NDY guidelines I discuss the opportunity with Sam. Several projects have been my Rotary club initiatives.

During my time in Sydney, I was very focussed on my fitness. We had a touch football team which was fun, but work at the gym was going strongly. I had a personal trainer and we both agreed that I should go in the 2005 City to surf race. I competed in 3 city to surfs, a half marathon and several 10K runs. Key to it all is putting in the training effort to run a time you are proud of and the run is the reward for months of training. Given I was 53 when this started, I was happy with my efforts. It was noticeable that I was not losing weight in this period despite a heavy training schedule and was disappointed in that aspect. In retrospect I now know had Cushing's at this stage and to not gain more weight than I did was an effort which I am now proud of.

Chapter 11. Various Locations 2007 to 2009

Given my intention to retire in 2009, it was time in 2007 to start looking for a replacement as Sydney Office Director. There was no heir apparent, so we put together a committee of five of our senior staff to run the office with me acting in an advisory and support role. It became clear that the appropriate person to run the office was James Henshaw. James was a Mechanical Engineer who had started as a graduate in the Melbourne Office and recently relocated to Sydney. He was very good with people and was well regarded by staff and clients. James came from a family of lawyers, so he had a good understanding of the issues we faced. He took over the role as Legal and Risk Director and I supported him particularly in matters which came to light during my time in the role. I was also consulted on some of the trickier problems where a detailed look at the problem was warranted. Often the people directly involved in the project underestimated the exposure we have.

During this period, I had the time to take on project work at the engineering level which I enjoyed greatly. NDY had an excellent relationship with Grocon, and both Tony Lukic and I knew Daniel Grollo quite well. They were considering taking on a high rise development in Brisbane. Early design work had been done, but there was concern at that the mechanical services design was not sufficiently developed to allow reliable prices to be obtained. Grocon wanted the concept design to be developed in 6 weeks, a very tight time frame given the size and complexity of the project.

Given the Sydney office was flat out at the time, this was a major task. I had many other duties so only a portion of my time could be devoted to the job. A task like this needs a very experienced engineer. By this time, Bill Drew (a mentor of mine) had long been retired and I asked him to help. He was still sharp as a tack and was a joy to work with as we put together the design. The major issue was that the previous work had failed to establish sufficient space for plant rooms, shafts and ductwork in the ceilings. The concept design was completed on time and Grocon were very pleased with the result.

This led to Grocon asking us to do a review of the mechanical design for the Oracle project on the Gold Coast. In particular, they were keen to identify cost savings. The design had been done by a competitor of ours whose Gold Coast Office was managed by Mark Bastin, an Engineer who had worked for me as a graduate in my days on the Gold Coast. We were unable to identify any substantial savings or errors. This was disappointing for Grocon, but I was pleased to see Mark had developed his skills.

I thought my presence in the Sydney office might diminish James' authority, so we looked elsewhere for opportunities to apply my talents. Melbourne office had recently lost several senior mechanical engineers

Chapter 11 – Various Locations 2007 to 2009

due mainly to relocations to other offices and were in desperate need of a leader. For the next several months I commuted to Melbourne to sort the situation out. I was impressed by the younger engineers who waded in. They needed more guidance.

A couple of projects were running into issues. One was the Myer store redevelopment. At the time this was the biggest department store in the world. It consisted of several old buildings joined together. Each of them had a different structure. The floor levels differed slightly in each building, requiring ramps. All in all, it was a real challenge for the coordination of ductwork and other services. We had changed staff several times due to the loss of senior staff in the office and had lost the confidence of the project manager and Builder. With the assistance of some inexperienced but enthusiastic engineers and my attendance at the project meetings, we were able to turn the situation around to the extent that we were waiting information from other parties to be able to complete the design.

Another project was a new building at the Victoria University. It included a facility which simulated high altitude training. This allowed training at an altitude of up to 3,000 m. It also required temperatures from -5 deg C to 40 deg C. The simulation of altitude was achieved by injection of nitrogen which reduced oxygen to the levels expected at high altitude. This equipment to do this was provided by a design and construct contractor. The control of temperature and humidity in the ranges sought required a very elaborate design which was provided. This job was successfully completed, and the room became a training facility for the Western Bulldogs AFL team.

In 2007, the world was in a construction boom and engineers and other technical staff were extremely difficult to find. We decided to join exhibition group which was focussed on obtaining engineering staff for Australian organisations. Exhibits were held in exhibition centres in Johannesburg, London and Manchester. I was required to be in London for the concept planning of the Stratford Shopping Centre, so we planned travel to suit the road show. NDY had government approval to sponsor staff to Australia. CEO Ian Hopkins and I manned the Johannesburg event. Retired director Don Miller helped me in Manchester. We were reasonably successful and, given we did not have to pay recruitment agent fees, it was financially worthwhile. Whilst we were somewhat nervous at the size of the boom, we were in, the size of the crash in 2008 was a surprise. The bigger the boom, the bigger the crash!

I was also asked to head up was the Nakheel Tall Tower in Dubai. NDY's London Office had been employed to proof engineer the design of the Mechanical and Electrical consultant. But the London office was overloaded at the time. At the same time, we were given notice by Nakheel's project managers that they were concerned with the work of the incumbent consultants and may require us to step in to handle the job. The project was planned to be 235 storeys high and over 1 km high. The building was circular with a diameter of 95 m. This would have been by far the tallest and largest commercial building ever built.

Chapter 11 – Various Locations 2007 to 2009

NDY were awarded the role on the recommendations of the project managers who were individuals we knew well. They had previously been with Multiplex in Melbourne and had worked closely with NDY, and particularly George Balales, a director of NDY with whom the project managers had enjoyed a close relationship on a previous project.

One key advantage in designing a tower of this height was our experience on the Eureka Tower in Melbourne, a very high-rise apartment tower. As buildings become higher, the traditional form of escape on fire alarm (walk down the fire stairs) becomes impractical. NDY were responsible for coming up with a concept which provided "safe havens" at various floors in the tower. People would have to descend a limited number of floors to reach the safe haven. The lifts were designed to continue operation during a fire and would carry the occupants down to the ground level. Eureka was the first building in the world to have such a design. It was an obvious requirement for the Nakheel Tower.

Our London Office was overloaded so it was agreed that the project would be transferred to Sydney, and I would be responsible for it. Nakheel then asked us to submit a proposal to take on the full role for design and contract administration. The project would require us to open an office in Dubai and staff it very quickly –about 30 staff would be required locally for the schematic design, with additional assistance provided remotely from other offices. The detailed design would require about 90 staff. The Tall Tower was surrounded by smaller (about 80 storeys) which may have also be added in our scope. The challenges of the project would make it difficult for us to take on other work, and this would put us in a precarious position should the project be abandoned which is far from unusual in such a project.

I worked closely with our CEO Ian Hopkins to prepare our offer. We decided we would submit a bid, with a fee set at a level which we thought covered our risk. The fee was accepted and so the planning for the new office started in earnest. We had a target date for the office to be opened in September 2008. I was available to arrive in July 2008. The project managers had worked with NDY's George Balalas in Melbourne and were keen to have him head up the job for NDY. George was tied up working on the South Australian Medical Research Institute. We committed George to be the Manager of the Dubai office in future stages and involved in a review role in the initial phase. I was to manage the office and hand over to George when he had completed his commitments in Adelaide. This put back my retirement plans, but it was a vital project for NDY and I was excited at the opportunity and felt I had had the experience to establish and manage the office required for the project.

Meanwhile assistance was required in London where we were documenting Stratford Shopping Centre. I had worked on preliminary stages of the project during previous visits to London. This is an enormous retail and entertainment complex adjacent the 2012 Olympic site. The developer was Westfield who we knew well in Australia, where we had worked for them on a series of projects. Given the location, it required multiple forms of transport, and the following were provided -:

- Tube station
- Bus interchange
- Overland rail
- Euro rail

When you arrived via public transport, the easiest route to access the Olympic Stadium was via the shopping centre.

The size of the project and the tightness of program demanded a large team, and I filled the role of mechanical team leader. The site was enormous, and this dictated many drawings per floor. Ducts and pipes crossed the joint in the drawings, which were being produced by different draughtspersons at different times and a key issue was to ensure that the sizes and flow rates were consistent in each drawing.

I also worked on the concept design for the refurbishment of The Angel Building in Islington. The original building air conditioning system was a ceiling mounted fan coil system. The developer was very keen to offer a state of the art system. Several alternatives were examined, and ultimately a displacement system was selected. A tiled floor was installed at say 300 mm above the concrete slab. Cool air at say 20 deg C was distributed through the false floor and flowed through grilles in the floor at low velocity. Cold air falls and by keeping the grille velocity low, a layer of cool air exists at low level. Where there is a heat source (say a person or a window) the heat induces an upward flow of air. The fact that we were supplying air at 20 deg C as compared with say 15 deg C in a conventional system provides the opportunity to save energy. In London, external temperatures are less than 20 deg C for much of the year and outside air can be used for cooling in lieu of a chiller.

During my stay in London, some more signs of Cushing's disease began to show. As well as being chronically tired I put on a lot of weight and acquired a "moon face" and "buffalo hump". I put this down to a reduction in the amount of exercise I was doing. Actually, I was going to the gym regularly and used to be a regular runner around the streets of the Barbican. From 2005 to 2007 I had been on a more stringent program to assist me in preparing for runs such as the City to Surf, Sydney half marathon and various 10 k runs.

I tore a few muscles and put this down to my lack of fitness. At the end of 2008. My blood pressure was high for the first time in my life. I was feeling unwell, and my sleep patterns were getting worse. I would wake up at 3:00 am and do the work which required communication with Australia – I still had significant corporate responsibilities. Overall my enthusiasm for the job outweighed my illness. Looking back, I don't think I could have endured my illness if I did not have such a challenging job.

At the end of my stint in London I was to head to Dubai. Deborah is a twin and has twin sisters a couple of years older. The older twin sisters share my birthday which

Chapter 11 – Various Locations 2007 to 2009

is 15th July. One of the older twins, Catherine was in London on a holiday with her husband David on 15th July 2008. We celebrated at Jamie Oliver's Restaurant Fifteen which is on the east side of London close to NDY's offices. We had a table on the lower floor. Deborah needed to go to the toilet and at the doorway there was a single step down to the bathroom level which is never a good idea. She missed the step and injured her foot badly. The waiter provided us with a complimentary bottle of French champagne. I could tell she was suffering because she did not enjoy the bubbles.

The next day she was still in great pain, and we went to accident and emergency at St Thomas' Hospital. Deborah had her foot x-rayed, and it showed a broken bone. It was put in plaster with the foot bent downward which I found strange. During my sporting activities I had observed that foot injuries require the foot to be bent upwards. The use of plaster seemed to be outdated. She was not seen by a doctor, the whole matter being dealt with by a nurse. All in all, I am certainly glad we have such a good health system in Australia.

The next day we flew from London to Dubai where I was to commence the establishment of the Dubai Office. Deborah was not able to get around on crutches, so we went to the American Hospital in Dubai. I don't think there is any American ownership, it is just a name. We waited for only 10 minutes before we were seen by a specialist doctor. He cut off the plaster, bandaged the foot bending upwards and provided a moon boot. We were able to hire a wheelchair at the hospital and head back to our hotel room. Through that and other experiences I found the health system in Dubai to be excellent.

Deborah was in a wheelchair for some time. You really notice the issues with handicapped access when you are handicapped yourself or are a carer for a handicapped person. The buildings in Dubai are built to international standards. Once you get out into the streets access got difficult. The amount of construction going on contributed to the problem.

Fortunately, I had no office and was working from our apartment which was in a high rise unit in Dubai Marina. I was able to help Deborah get around, a favour that she would pay back many times over in future years. I began to get to know the participants in the Tall Tower project. I had not dealt with the project managers who were employed directly by Nakheel to manage the project, but they had previous favourable experience with NDY. That was the key factor in NDY winning the job.

The client's representative for building services was Neil Woodcock who had considerable experience in England and the UK. Things are done differently around the world and Neil's knowledge and experience was to be invaluable in our work. One local custom for expats was Friday Breakfasts which were a feature for many of the international hotels. They featured an amazing variety and quantity of food and unlimited French champagne. Friday is the sabbath in the middle east and Sunday is a work day.

The Architects for the project were Woods Bagot, an Australian company. NDY had worked with them on many

Chapter 11 – Various Locations 2007 to 2009

occasions. I had over the years developed a friendship with David Tregonning who was at that time the world CEO for the company. Prior to taking that role he was responsible for the Sydney office. He was also a regular on our Boxing Day cruise for the start of the Sydney to Hobart yacht race.

Whilst I did not know the individuals working on the job for Woods Bagot, I am sure they would have received positive vibes from their colleagues. As time went on it became apparent that Woods Bagot had picked the A team for the project and they really did a great job.

The Structural Engineers were WPS from New York, and we had no experience working with them. Rider Hunt were the Quantity Surveyors and we had worked with them on a multitude of projects around the world.

I had been working on recruiting for some time. I wanted to have a senior person or two in each discipline who was known and trusted. This meant transferring in key people from other offices. This was at a time just before the Global Financial Crisis when the property market was overheated, and engineers were very hard to get. I was very grateful to my fellow directors who provided staff in all the key roles.

People who were transferred to Dubai included:

- Geoff Cullen who had been a director in the Perth prior to retiring, upon which he had continued part time employment. Besides being an excellent engineer, Geoff is a lot of fun to be with and was an ideal personality to be involved in a start-up office.

- Peter Koulos, whom I had employed as a graduate. Since then, Peter worked several years in the Sydney office, then transferred to London.
- Frank Bakker who was a fire engineer. These days it is acceptable to provided design solutions which meet the intent of the Building Code. Each clause of the code specifies a "deemed to comply" method and provides the intent of the particular clause. Fire Engineers require a specific degree. Frank had been a Fire Officer with the Canberra fire brigade and then studied for his degree before joining NDY.
- Isaac Coker, an Associate Director and Mechanical Engineer from our London Office. Isaac was of African parentage and was a very gentle and loyal friend to all of us.
- Lesley Giblin, my PA from the Sydney office. Before leaving for Dubai, Lesley had the task of arranging transport, visas and accommodation for the people going to Dubai. She went to Dubai to set up our administrative systems and take care of the incoming staff.

I was again called upon Bill Drew to assist. He was unable to come to Dubai but could work from the Sydney office. We also assigned quite a bit of work to other offices.

The office start up was planned for September 2008. I needed to attend the NDY Directors and Manager's meeting which was held during August in Noosa on Queensland's Sunshine Coast. A key issue for the office opening was the effect Ramadan would have on our planning. Whilst it was possible to buy alcoholic beverages

Chapter 11 – Various Locations 2007 to 2009

in some of the Emirates, these were closed for Ramadan. The thought of 20 very thirsty engineers not being able to get a drink was most concerning. The office may well have failed at that point. The solution was the Barracuda run. The Barracuda Hotel in Ajman sold alcohol. Given the lack of sales tax in the Emirates, it may well have had the cheapest grog in the world. I hired a Toyota Yaris and drove up to the Hotel. The Yaris was packed to the gunnels with a variety of beverages, and I headed back to Dubai. Ajman is surrounded by Sharjah where it is illegal to possess alcohol. It only takes about 10 minutes of very careful driving to get through Sharjah.

I arrived back at the apartment and loaded the grog into the Apartment. I may have overdone the quantity a little. The next day I left for Noosa and the meetings. A golf day was an essential part of our meetings, so we teed off at Noosa Springs. My old friend Don Miller was in my foursome. Don was known to hit the occasional ball astray and I was foolish enough to be standing ahead of him, albeit well into the rough. Don hit a low hook which zeroed in on my left leg just above the ankle on the inside.

Within an hour I was bruised from my groin to the tips of my toes. This seemed totally disproportionate to the injury, which was not all that painful. I visited a doctor, but there was nothing which could be done for it. I needed to fly back to Dubai, so went to the local hospital to have an ultrasound. The blood flow was OK, and I was good to fly.

Whilst in Noosa I received a phone call from the Filipino lady who managed our apartment. "You have "alcohols" in your apartment" I replied "Yes I do". She told me "You are not allowed to have alcohols in your lease". The lease did not actually say anything about alcohol, but it was probably illegal in Dubai. Apartment leases were hard to come by, so I did not argue the point. She insisted I remove the alcohols that day. It took a while for her to understand that I was in Australia and could not do that. Eventually we agreed I could have a few more days. When I returned to Dubai, I was able to store the booze with friends.

A week or two later, I noticed my golf ball injury had gone a blood red colour The impact had not broken the skin, but it was clear something untoward was happening. I went to the local GP who lanced the injury, then was shocked at the hole that opened up. I had a hematoma which extended down to the bone. The doctor packed the wound, then injected me with penicillin. I had injections daily for a couple of weeks until the danger of infection had passed. No doubt this extraordinary injury was related to my yet to be diagnosed Cushing's disease.

I could not wear a normal shoe for a couple of months, so wore Arabian style sandals with socks along with my business apparel. I thought I might start a new trend, but no one else had the fashion sense to adopt the look.

I kept up an exercise routine using the gym in the apartment complex despite the ankle injury. It was much too hot in Dubai to go for a run outside. My weight continued to rise and I developed sciatica. I discovered many years later that this was caused by compression fractures to L4 and L5. I have no memory of having any

Chapter 11 – Various Locations 2007 to 2009

incident that would cause such an injury and believe this to be caused by Cushing's Disease which causes osteoporosis. As the osteoporosis was well developed in 2008, I think the disease must have been in place for at least 5 years by then

On top of that, my chronic tiredness worsened, and I was feeling unwell and could not put my finger on a reason.

My professional responsibilities were considerable. I believe that I had the best job in the world for a building services consultant at that time. I had been prominent in securing the job for NDY which reflected very favourably on the company. Then I was responsible for setting up the organisation whilst coordinating the building services on the biggest and tallest building in the world. That gave me the impetus to push my illness aside.

The site was in a completely undeveloped area not far from my unit in Dubai Marina. The site was basically a desert. It was part of a long term plan to develop the land around a yet to be constructed canal. The canal would be in a U shape connecting to the Arabian gulf in two locations and each of the three legs on the U would be 25 km.

We were offered office space in on site sheds which were done quite well. The client provided the accommodation free of cost. We were the only consultants who had their entire Tall Tower Team on site. Other consultants had few if any staff on site. Since we had only the one project in Dubai, there was no issue with this arrangement. Besides, I love a bargain!

On arrival, our staff were put up in a newly finished hotel in a new suburb close to our development site. It was staggering to see a whole suburb complete with houses, apartment buildings, retail precincts, transport links community facilities and the like all built at the one time. This was occurring in multiple locations around Dubai at that time.

I developed an understanding of how these projects work financially. Firstly, understand that most of Dubai is basically owned by the government which is effectively the Royal Family (Sheiks). The land is worthless desert. When a new development is planned, one of the Sheiks' development companies plans a "signature building", typically a lavish tall building. It also plans and constructs waterways, roads and infrastructure such as power, telecommunications, water, stormwater, sewerage and district chilled water schemes which are owned by the Sheik's companies. If one was to do an economic analysis of the signature building on a stand alone basis, the return on investment would be poor. The value of the land adjacent the signature tower is enhanced greatly. This land is sold off the third party developers from places such as India and the nearby Arab countries, who develop properties as guided by the master plan prepared by the Sheiks' companies.

The approach is not dissimilar to that seen in Western Countries where a developer will finance and build a golf course to enhance the value of the adjacent residential land.

The utilities companies were unable to keep up with the pace of development. Power might have to be provided initially by generators. Sewerage was held temporarily

Chapter 11 – Various Locations 2007 to 2009

in holding tanks whilst the pipes and treatment plants were being completed. Tanker trucks would pump out the holding tanks and transport this to a sewerage treatment plant. The tankers might have to wait 24 hrs or so to be able to empty. It was not unknown for the drivers to illegally empty the waste into a stormwater line. That line would discharge untreated sewerage into the Arabian Gulf. Of course, the authorities applied significant penalties to drivers caught doing this.

When I was in Dubai, there was, incredibly, a shortage of diesel and petrol. The Government had in place a limit on the price it would pay the oil companies for oil. The price of oil had escalated well above that level, so the oil companies ceased to sell to the Government. Tanker trucks were queued up waiting for fuel. The international press loved the irony and photos of the tanker queues were featured around the world. It was embarrassing for the Government.

And how was the problem fixed? Firstly, tanker drivers had to obtain a permit to obtain fuel. They could be fined if they lined up for fuel without a permit, which strangely were very hard to get. In addition, it became illegal for the tankers to wait in line for more than a few hours.

That brings me to the subject of Dubai red tape. There were books written on it however the books were of little use because the rules changed before a book could be written and published. One of the ways a company of our intended size can go is to employ a sponsor. Sponsors were all Emiratis. They were there to smooth the way for a foreign business to open in Dubai. Dubai does not have any taxes, but this seemed a convenient way to transfer funds from foreign companies to the locals.

The company could not open a bank account until we registered a business. To register a business, it must have a bank account. NDY Dubai survived on Credit Cards. I personally survived on my Australian bank accounts, credit cards and ATM's.

To operate as Engineers, we required a license from the Dubai Municipal Council. This required us to submit details online for assessment. Then an interview was arranged with a council officer, myself and our sponsor. The council officer raised new requirements which we went away and dealt with. Then another meeting was arranged with a different Council officer who had different requirements. This was repeated several times and I decided a new approach was needed.

I had employed Mohammed (Mo) Ali as a graduate engineer in the Sydney office. He was a very good engineer who handled himself very well with clients. Mo had transferred to the London office. He was currently working for NDY in Abu Dhabi working onsite on a major project. Mo was of Lebanese parentage and spent his early life in Dubai until his family emigrated to Australia where he went to high school and university. He spoke fluent Arabic.

Our sponsor was not available to attend the meeting. Most of the discussion was in Arabic which the Dubai Council Officers were more comfortable with. Mo was able to answer most of the questions with the occasional

Chapter 11 – Various Locations 2007 to 2009

one translated and handled by me. We were advised verbally that we would be registered and received written confirmation a couple of days later.

The government was quite invasive in the way they kept an eye on the immigrants. Employers were required to advise the Government when an employee was terminated. The Government would contact the employee and required the employee to obtain another job or leave the country. The banks were also advised. If the person did not have permanent employment the bank would demand immediate repayment of any loans the person had. Failure to repay would result in imprisonment, which was terminated when the loan was repaid. This led to the well known situation where people would leave their cars at the airport on their way out.

I had a rental car. When I received my work permit, I was contacted by the rental company and advised I could not continue to rent the car unless I obtained a local license. Big Brother was certainly watching.

We commenced work on the Tall Tower project. The greatest difficult we initially faced was the Air Conditioning of the office floors which occupied the lower 50 floors of the tower. Our client favoured a variable volume system with a central air handling plant. Such a system has air handling plant located every 20 to 30 floors and air is supplied via vertical ducts to each floor.

The structure for the building featured a 60 m diameter, 1.5 m thick cylinder extending from the foundation the full height of the building. This was required to withstand wind forces which are considerable on a tower of this height. The cylinder could be penetrated for doors, ducts, pipes and conduits provided the holes in the structure were spread out and not concentrated. Unfortunately, the preliminary Architectural design had located most of the lifts (and there were 169 lifts in the building) immediately inside the structural cylinder. There were corridors through the cylinder which constituted large penetrations. The penetrations required for the air conditioning could not be accommodated in the available space.

At the first meeting to work through this issue, NDY's Geoff Cullen wore a Tee shirt he had made up for the event. It featured a cartoon character in the form of a large drill. The caption read "The Penetrator". The humour was appreciated by all. As a result of that meeting, the Architects redesigned the core of the building relocating the lift away from the structural cylinder where possible and located the vertical air conditioning shafts immediately inside the cylinder. This enabled our duct penetrations to be located away from the door penetrations, where they could be structurally accommodated. They did a remarkable job in short time and the team was able to quickly establish a viable design for the office floors.

The design of Tall Towers is driven by the wind forces. The horizontal force tries to push the building over. The structural engineer must design the structure and foundations of the building to resist these forces. To put it in perspective, the wind force acting on the "leeward" side

Chapter 11 – Various Locations 2007 to 2009

of the Nakheel Tall Tower was 10 times the force due to the weight of the building, giving a total force of 11 times the gravitational force. On the "windward" side of the building, there was an upwards force due to wind of 10 times the gravitational force, offset slightly by the gravitational force to give a nett upward force of 9 times the gravitational force. So the structure had to simultaneously counter a major downward force on one side of the building and a major upward force on the other side.

All tall towers use some sort of trick to lower the wind forces on the building. The most common is reducing the size of the tower at the upper floors of the building, as per the Burj Khalif Tower in Dubai which is, at 828 m, the highest building in the world. The Nakheel Tall Tower used a different trick. The building was actually 4 separate buildings, each of them a quadrant, with a cross shaped breezeway which relieved the pressures on the building. At about 30 floor intervals, there were 4 complete "satellite" floors which tied the structure together. In some segments of the building, the quadrants were hotel suites, in others apartments.

High rise buildings only became feasible when Elisha Otis invented lifts in the mid 19th century. The Tall Towers of today are reliant on modern high speed double deck lifts which operate at about 10 m/sec. To gain the speed advantage, lifts need to bypass most floors. In the Nakheel Tall tower, double deck high speed lifts shuttled passengers from the ground floor directly to each group of satellite floors, serving the upper two floors in each satellite. These floors would include spaces such as reception, cafes, restaurants, bars and gymnasiums. Four sets of local lifts would be provided, one for each quadrant of the building. The two upper satellite floors were linked by escalators.

The lower two satellite floors were building services floors and very much the province of NDY. The pressure able to be withstood by piping is such that, at the most, a piping system could only serve the height of two satellite sections of the building, with a preference to serve only one. The domestic water supply had storage tanks at each satellite with water pumped into the tanks from below, and out of the tanks to above. A similar principal was adopted for the fire sprinkler system and the hydrant and hose reel system.

The situation became more tricky with chilled water required for air conditioning. When chilled water goes from one vertical stage to another, it must go through a heat exchanger which isolates the "water in" side from the "water out" side but allows heat transfer between them. Each time a heat exchanger is used, the water temperature on the water going out is about 0.75 deg C higher than the water going in. There were 7 sets of satellite floors. If we were to put heat exchangers at every set of satellite floors, the temperature rise between the chillers at ground level and the top of the building would be 5.25 deg C. This would dictate the need for using glycol (an anti-freeze) in the chillers which was undesirable and inefficient. We chose instead to only have heat exchangers at every second set of satellite floors and allowing for the high pressure on pipework.

Chapter 11 – Various Locations 2007 to 2009

Bill Drew then identified a further issue. The barrier between the two water circuits in the heat exchangers could fail. This would subject the lower circuit to double the pressure intended and would cause the system to fail. That would cause a failure in the heat exchanger below, thus setting up a "daisy chain' of failures and causing considerable damage to equipment as well as water damage to the building. After a few days of contemplation and checking facts with heat exchanger manufacturers, we worked out we could prevent this by providing relief vents on all heat exchangers which relieved the pressure in the event of heat exchange failure.

This was one of many issues to be solved for the Tall Tower. The strangest problem of all was reverse stack effect. I'll start by explaining stack effect which was first noticed in tall buildings in the colder regions of the USA and Canada. Imagine a chimney the height of a building. It is winter and a fire is lit at the base of the chimney. What will occur is a rise of temperature in the chimney. The heat causes a build-up of pressure which forces the air to flow upwards through the chimney. The pressure potentially created is a function of the height of the building times the temperature difference between inside the building and outside the building.

Reverse stack effect occurs in tall buildings during summer in hot climates. Cold air falls and creates a high pressure in the lower floors of the building and a low pressure at the top of the building. The combination of the height of the building at 1km and outside temperature of 47 deg C would cause very high reverse stack pressures significantly more than any high rise building ever built.

Several different remedies were devised: -

At the pedestrian entries, there would be a revolving door linked by a passage to a second revolving door. At goods vehicle entries with an ante room. A vehicle arriving to the site would enter the ante room from outside and the doors would be closed to form a sealed room. A damper would open to the inside of the ante room equalise the pressure. The internal doors would then open allowing the vehicle to enter the building.

Car park entry would be open to the atmosphere. An ante room would be provided for pedestrian access operating as described above. In the tower, access would be needed outside for maintenance purposes. Ante rooms would be provided.

The longer lift shafts and fire escape stairs would be air conditioned which negates the reverse cycle effect.

The location of chillers and cooling of them required some thought. On most projects, we would put them on the roof. On the tall tower, the roof was at 1 km and the access would require an ante room. Winds at the that level would preclude maintenance frequently. The hoisting of parts to and from the roof also presented a problem. So plant was located at low level.

The cooling water was best sourced from the canal which was yet to be built. The canal would need to provide cooling water for a great number of buildings. Therefore the authorities required the water returned to the canal to

Chapter 11 – Various Locations 2007 to 2009

be no warmer than the water taken from the canal. Geoff Cullen was assigned the task of solving this problem. He borrowed a solution from the power industry. The canal water would be used to cool the chillers. The water flowing out of the chillers would pass through the cooling towers before being returned to the canal. Heat exchangers would isolate the chillers from the salt water of the canal.

The published design temperature for Dubai is 47 deg C. This is the temperature which is used as the basis for air conditioning calculations. Some people were sceptical that this temperature was low. The reason was that local laws required building sites to close if the temperature exceeded 47 deg C. The daily temperature often got to 47 deg C but rarely exceeded it.

Bill Drew sourced data available on the internet based on a series of weather balloons which had been released from Abu Dhabi airport. These transmitted the temperature until they travelled out of range. Air conditioning theory allows the design temperature to be reduced at high levels. This would reduce the required capacity of the air conditioning systems in the upper floors of the building substantially. However, the data from the weather balloons seemed to contradict the theory and in fact recorded high level temperatures above ground level temperatures. Bill wrote a program to analyse the data. What was happening became clear. In the day the ground would heat up. The air at high level would not be affected as much. At night the ground would cool down and the high level air would not cool down as much. We satisfied ourselves that the air conditioning theory was correct.

A further consideration was how to manage the microprocessor control systems. This project had a construction period of 10 years. If we followed the normal process and called tenders for microprocessor controls at the same time the other building services were tendered, the equipment would be out of date by several generations when it was installed. In consultation with our client the team devised a way of delaying the controls tenders until late in the construction program.

The electrical supply required was to be 1200 MW, sufficient for a township. High voltage power was reticulated up the tower, with two substations provided at each set of satellite floors. High voltage generators located at low level also served all transformers, thus providing standby and emergency power. Emergency and power circuits were fed from both substations at each satellite level.

Come the first Tuesday of November and time for Melbourne Cup. We were on site by that time, so decided to celebrate in normal Aussie fashion with NDY putting on the party. The Cup was run at 7:30 am local time. We invited all the other consultants and the Nakheel team. The site office also had cleaners and security guards who were also invited. They were Moslem Pakistanis and so we had to be careful how we handled it. Deborah bought some local items including chocolates and shishas as prizes in the sweep. Tickets were given away, gambling being illegal in Dubai. The internet fell over and we missed the race live but managed to see a replay. A few discreet bubbles were consumed prior to work starting.

Chapter 11 – Various Locations 2007 to 2009

The world financial crisis was happening by this time. The Sheiks had to abandon most of their projects under pressure from the banks but were determined to go ahead with the Tall Tower. Then they advised that the project would be delayed. I could see the writing on the wall and stopped the planned arrival of staff into the country. I had a real concern that the project would be abandoned. I sought involvement with several projects and made bids for several. None of the projects went ahead and the market was effectively dead.

While we were flat out on the Nakheel Tall Tower, our London Office was approached regarding a "mega project" in Bahrain. A team was being assembled and NDY was asked to come on board as Building Services Engineers. The team certainly had good credentials, so we agreed to become involved. The project was being undertaken by the Bahrain Royal family and the person organising the project was a retired General from Turkey. I shall refer to him as the "General". As well as being the Project Director, he would be the agent responsible for obtaining the necessary permits for each of the various members of the design team.

The project was to be carried out on islands (existing and yet to be created) in the Arabian Sea which would be linked to each other and the mainland by a series of causeways, a similar concept to the islands created in Dubai. For NDY it was a dilemma. On the one hand, we were very exposed if the Nakheel Tall Tower failed to go ahead. On the other, we had our hands full coping with the Nakheel job, and handling two such massive jobs in a brand new office was a daunting prospect.

The General was calling the shots. He was also requiring each of the design team companies to employ him to act as their agent. Effectively this would be similar to the situation in Dubai and not unusual in the Middle East. Some of the other members of the team had already been registered in this manner, so it seemed above board. I personally did not think the Bahrain project was likely to go ahead and we should not spend the funds being sought for registration. The consensus of the NDY Board was that we should go with the project.

A meeting was called in Bahrain and all the design team members were required to attend. We were required to pay a fee of UK£10,000 in cash to the General when we arrived in Dubai. That exceeds the amount which can be carried out of Dubai, and I was not prepared to do that. Arrangements were made to withdraw the funds from a bank in Bahrain on my arrival which all worked. The General arranged to meet us on the air side of customs and immigration which he did. That indicates he carried some clout.

We had a worthwhile series of meetings and then departed. The job raised its head a few times after that but effectively died. To this day I don't know whether it was a pipe dream or a victim of the Global Financial Crisis.

I returned to Australia for the Christmas/New Year break and on 23rd December I was advised by telephone that the project was officially abandoned. I wanted to advise the staff in person of the situation before they heard it on the grapevine. I cut my holidays short and flew back, arriving

Chapter 11 – Various Locations 2007 to 2009

early on Sunday 28th December 2008. Sundays are not a holiday in the Emirates, and I had arranged to have a staff meeting, at which I advised them of the situation and that the office would be winding back to a few people. I then had a private meeting with each of them to discuss their future. NDY could offer a role in another office for most of them, but a few wanted to work in the Middle East in which case we negotiated a redundancy package. All in all, I think it went as well as possible. It was a terrible day for me.

Our fees remained unpaid, and arrangements were put in place to pay these. We kept the office open with minimal staff, including me. We continued to chase work but there was none available. It was a particularly frustrating few months and without the thrill of a massive project, I felt the weight of the still to be diagnosed Cushing's Disease. It took a considerable period, but our fees were paid in full, well after I left Dubai. I think we were fortunate in that, if we had been working for a developer in Australia in similar circumstances, we would have been left high and dry.

The stark difference in how I felt when the job was going ahead full steam, as compared to how I felt after it fell over, makes me realise how lucky I was to have such a challenge in my life.

During the time in Dubai, Deborah and I made the decision to rent our Sydney home and occupy a unit we held at Main Beach on the Gold Coast, closer to our families. We had the intention to retire on the Gold Coast after I had completed my responsibilities in Dubai. Deborah split her time between the Gold Coast and Dubai.

Chapter 12. Gold Coast 2009 to 2013

I arrived back on the Gold Coast and took holidays which I badly needed. It also provided time for the company to sort out what, if anything, I should be doing for the company in the future. If I was to retire at that stage I would have done so without regret. The decision was made that we needed to diversify away from commercial property, and I was appointed Director for Industrial and Infrastructure. Commercial property was hit hard world-wide in the GFC and in previous downturns. Banks stopped lending to the sector. On the other hand, Governments increased funding of infrastructure. I was keen to take on the challenge.

In late 2009, I suffered from Deep Vein Thrombosis (blood clotting) following a flight home from Hawaii where Deborah and I had enjoyed a holiday. It was in the left leg and had spread to both lungs. It was some 3 weeks after the flight, and I was in Sydney for the week working when I noticed a swelling in my left leg and thought it might have been a recurrence of the hematoma from the golf injury. I had from a golf ball impact. I caught a taxi at 3:00 am to A and E at Royal North Shore Hospital. The were very few patients waiting and the triage nurse saw me immediately. I told her about my golf ball injury. She asked me "Have you had a long flight recently?" to which I replied, "From

Chapter 12 – Gold Coast 2009 to 2013

Honolulu but it was 3 weeks ago". She said, "You seem a little breathless". I hadn't realised it, but she was correct. I was immediately put into an emergency bed and given an injection of clexane, a blood thinner which acts immediately. Later that morning I underwent ultrasounds which verified I had a DVT in my leg and Pulmonary Embolism in both lungs. Cushing's disease increases the risk of clotting, so may well have been a factor.

Deborah was on her way to Sydney that morning and I managed to phone her before she caught her flight. Having been a flight attendant she was aware of the risks of clotting whereas I was quite ignorant. She was concerned much more than I was. I spent 3 days in hospital, during which I started taking Warfarin. On discharge from hospital, Deborah and I stayed with our long term friends, John and Deborah Darragh at Balgowlah Heights. I was referred to home nursing by a nurse at the hospital who described me as a "delightful elderly gentleman". At age 56 I wasn't sure whether this was a compliment or not. The home nursing services attended to me, giving me blood tests to check my warfarin doses and clexane injections while my warfarin levels built up. I learned how to self-inject, a skill which was to be required many times in the future.

A couple of days after my discharge, I was suffering pain in my stomach and reported back to Royal North Shore. I was admitted to emergency and was in a bed with a label "donated by the Rotary Club of Balgowlah" which was my old club in Sydney. Sometimes what comes around goes around. At the time they found no cause for the problem. Since then, a similar thing had happened several times due to internal bleeding. I now know I can't tolerate clexane at the normal levels prescribed and need to have about half dosage. It is a very powerful blood thinner.

Deborah and I headed back to the Gold Coast once things were under control.

My previous experience in the Sydney Office had included some involvement with vehicle and train tunnel services, which included ventilation, electrical and lighting, fire suppression, security and information technology. We had been successful in providing these services for the Tugun tunnel which was built to allow extension of the Gold Coast Airport runway.

Tunnel projects are few in number and very large in value. The business challenge is to be able to staff them at relatively short notice and then absorb the staff back into other projects as the tunnel project is completed. Staff needed to be able to swap from infrastructure projects to commercial jobs. This took time to develop, but we increased our foothold on tunnel work. These days, the company is one of the leading practices in this area.

IN 2010, I identified Rail Consultancy as a major opportunity. The problem was NDY had limited experience in that area – we had done mechanical and electrical services for stations and some work on train tunnel ventilation, but had no experience in rolling stock, maintenance facilities, or electrification.

I did not think it practical to acquire the skills within the company and began a search for a company we could

Chapter 12 – Gold Coast 2009 to 2013

develop a joint venture arrangement with. What I was looking for was:

- A company which did not currently operate in Australia. NDY had something to offer to such a company.
- A company which offered services in the mechanical and electrical areas and could provide "technology transfer" to NDY.
- A well respected company.
- A company of moderate size. I thought a large company would be likely to use us to gain entry to the Australian market, then branch out independently.

My search led me to LTK Engineering Services, headquartered in Philadelphia, Pennsylvania USA. They were a company of about 300 staff. Their biggest area of operation was rolling stock. By way of explanation, rolling stock are the locomotives and carriages which make up a train. Most people think these are a standard vehicle a manufacturer produces, and a rail company purchases. In fact, every rail company and rail network has unique needs, and the rolling stock is very specific. In addition, they designed electrification, maintenance facilities, refurbishment of rolling stock and had a leading edge simulation program to analyse performance of rail networks. Like NDY, they specialised in the mechanical/electrical side of things.

I sent several emails to LTK, with very little response and thought things were going nowhere. Deborah and I had a cruise planned departing from Fort Lauderdale, so I asked LTK's President George Dorshimer if he would like me to meet with him. He agreed, so I diverted my flights to Philly and had a couple of days there. It was the original capital of the USA after the War of Independence. It was also the location of the Declaration of Independence. Many of the historic buildings from that era are still in place.

I spent a few days absorbing the atmosphere of the place. It was the home of Benjamin Franklin and his post office still exists and operates. Old Ben was the author of the very wise statement *"Beer is proof that God loves us and wants us to be happy."* Plus the Liberty Bell and various museums.

LTKs Offices were at Ambler, a suburb of Philadelphia about 30 mins train ride from the city. It is much like a village and the biggest building is LTK's Headquarters. I attended a meeting with their shareholders. George Dorshimer gave a presentation on LTK, and I one on NDY. I think what worked for us all was the cultural fit between the two organisations.

We were both traditional engineering practices, with shareholders also the managers. We were both reasonably conservative. We are at the leading edge in our areas of expertise. LTK had never opened an office outside of North America. What NDY had to offer was office space and support, a good relationship with potential clients in the rail industry and some support technically. We also had a far bigger international operation. LTK provided the expertise.

George and Chris Lawlor (CFO) visited Australia and I accompanied them around the country, and we met

Chapter 12 – Gold Coast 2009 to 2013

with the various rail authorities. Meetings were held between the two companies to work out the basis of the joint venture agreement and an agreement on day to day operation.

Dominic de Brito was assigned by LTK and was appointed as Managing Director of NDY LTK. It became apparent that Dom was being groomed for greater things at LTK which eventually turned out to be appointment as President of the company upon George's retirement. Dom reported to me on a day-to-day basis, and I learned a little about rail design. He had an amazing work ethic. I would review reports and whilst I was not competent to comment technically, I could ask for clarifications on issues a client may be interested in. I also interpreted American into English.

NDYLTK Pty Ltd was licensed to provide services in most countries around the world. Our first job was for a Chinese rolling stock manufacturer to help them prepare a tender for equipment required in South Africa. The bid was unsuccessful, but our fees were fully paid.

The JV company had a major win in Victoria. We were selected to supply software and provide support and training to Yarra Trams, the metro system, and the overland rail. This enabled us to establish an office in Melbourne. We also picked up work in NSW for light rail in Sydney. We employed Australian staff in Sydney and Melbourne.

I valued the association with LTK and became firm friends with George, Chris and Dom.

Some time after I retired from NDY, a decision was made to sell NDY to a NASDAQ listed company. The joint venture agreement covered such a situation. LTK had the first call to purchase NDYLTK Pty Ltd and they did.

I was contacted by LTK on the occasion of the 100-year anniversary of their company in 2021. The following article appeared in their staff newsletter: -

Dennis O'Brien holds a special place in the history of LTK.
"He's the only non-LTK employee to ever be inducted onto the Wall of Fame," said George Dorshimer, past President of the firm.
And with good reason: Without O'Brien's vision and hard work, LTK would have never partnered with Norman Disney and Young (NDY) to form NDYLTK, and would most likely have never expanded to Australia.
O'Brien retired in 2013, and now lives in the Gold Coast in Australia with his wife Deborah and trusty daschund, Red.
But in 2008, he was the Deputy CEO for NDY's International Group and busy pursuing a huge project, which unfortunately fell through. However, as is often the case, when one window closes, another opens. In this case, it was an opportunity that led to the NDYLTK partnership.
"I was in Dubai setting up a new NDY organization to provide consultant services for the construction of the Nakheel Tower. It would have been the first building in the world over 1,000-meters high. Of course, in 2008 the global financial crisis [GFC] hit, and while the sheiks would have dearly loved to build their pride-and-joy, the banks reined them in and they were unable to do so. So, I had to wind up that operation, and from there we asked

Chapter 12 – Gold Coast 2009 to 2013

ourselves, 'OK, what do we do next?' It took a while to re-orient ourselves and we decided that we really needed to diversify and not be so reliant on commercial construction because it had basically slowed down worldwide.

"So, I was given the task of working out how we could diversify the firm. We looked at all the various little niches, but rail was the big one in Australia because there was so much rail work being planned and there had been an increased concentration on it in view of the economic downturn. There was no way we could get into rail from where we were. We didn't have the knowledge, so I started hunting around to see if there was a firm that might be a good fit with us. Most were megafirms, and I didn't think a relationship like that would work. There were some that already competed with us in building services and we thought that, if we invited them to Australia, there was a high probability that they would set up and become competition.

"I had never heard of LTK prior to finding them on the internet, but we didn't see any other firm that was as good a match for us. From what I could see, LTK was a firm very similar to our own in outlook and the way it operated. LTK was mechanical-electrical, not civil-structural as we are. It was similar to us in size – LTK might have had 300 employees and we had 400 to 450. And, geographically, LTK hadn't expanded much, and we had. We had offices and good relationships with various governments that we could use to introduce LTK.

"I contacted LTK in April of 2010. My wife and I travel a lot, and it so happened we were going to Fort Lauderdale for a cruise. I got George on the phone and said, 'I'm on my way [to the US], would you like me to come along and have a talk. He was very favorable to that, and I think we hit it off straightaway.

Dorshimer remembers O'Brien as being resolute in his belief that a partnership would benefit both firms.

"He was persistent because he thought we were the right partner for him," Dorshimer said. "We were skeptical – well, I was skeptical and some were dead-set against it. We had a four-hour meeting with him, and by the end of it he had convinced us that it was worth further exploration.

"I ended up taking an exploratory trip to Australia in August. Dennis took me around and we made a joint assessment of what we could do and what we couldn't do. So that's how I got to know him. I travelled all over Australia with him in 2010. The following year we made the decision to set up the new company and the rest is history. Dominic ended up going over and he built the company into a solid success. It's still a success, albeit all of it is now under Hatch."

According to DiBrito, it's O'Brien who deserves a lot of the credit.

"He was the individual with the vision and the tenacity to make Australia happen," said DiBrito. "He wasn't the CEO at NDY, but he was probably the most influential person within the organization on an operational, day-to-day basis. He had the vision to try new things and move the company in different directions. And, he was a great host. When I flew to Australia for the second time, it was to bring my wife, Kim, down to see if I could convince her to live there. Dennis saw the importance of that and invited us to use his boat as our hotel for the week we were in Queensland – knowing that was about the most significant thing he could do to convince my wife, who is an avid scuba diver, to move to Australia. That's Dennis move!"

Chapter 12 – Gold Coast 2009 to 2013

> *DiBrito, of course, ended up moving to Australia where he got to know O'Brien better than most.*
>
> *"I think something people probably don't necessarily remember, or know, about Dennis is that he was the force behind NDY's charitable trust program, which exists today. It's an employee-directed foundation that gives to charity. He developed it, then stepped away and let the employees manage it. We were actually very impressed with that and I think that influenced LTK's Volunteer Time Off policy and some of the other things that we've done.*
>
> *"Dennis is a great guy. His efforts coordinating the partnership are the reason that LTK Australia exists, and the reason he ended up on the Wall of Fame."*

I very much valued my association with LTK and consider it a highlight of my career. I had decided to sell my shareholding in NDY at the end of the 2012/13 financial year. Thereafter I would work as needed on a part time basis.

In the lead up to my retirement, I was very conscious that I needed to think seriously about what I intended to do in the future. I have a wide range of interests but was concerned that my as yet undiagnosed health concerns may preclude some of these. So, I thought in terms of "alternative futures". These included:
1. Living on the Gold Coast. Deborah and I believe it to be the best place in the world.
2. Working from home on a part or full-time basis for NDY.
3. Taking up a Project Management position.
4. Golf a couple of times a week.
5. Boating - we had a 12m cruiser moored at the Southport Yacht club a short walk from home.

6. Taking up bridge. I had learned to play on the various cruises we had been on and thought I could become a reasonable player.
7. Volunteering with the local surf club
8. Increased community work, with Rotary and perhaps in other endeavours.

As it turned out, these what actually happened was
1. We are on the Gold Coast and love our life here
2. I worked for several years part time for NDY, ending in about 2017
3. Not taken up
4. Played golf until about 2020 when the pain in my left leg and foot became unbearable
5. I could not manage the boat and reluctantly sold it.
6. I have taken up bridge but recent hospitalisations have limited my ability to attend.
7. Deterioration in my health precluded this.
8. I have stepped up my contributions to Rotary considerably.

In 2011 the Penthouse in our apartment building came up for sale and we were able to purchase it and moved in. We also had an architect draw up plans for a renovation. There were some issues with the original design and the general condition of the apartment was not good. My health had continued to deteriorate to the extent that the original renovation plans had a handicapped lift between the two floors of the penthouse. Given my poor health, we decided to defer the renovation.

My health had deteriorated further by the end of 2012. I had to pull out of trips planned to NZ and Melbourne.

Chapter 12 – Gold Coast 2009 to 2013

At the time I was heavily involved with writing our OH&S system along with Laura Esperanza from the Melbourne Office who was good enough to come up to the Gold Coast where we worked together on the system which was later given third party accreditation.

Deborah and I had decided to sell our Sydney House and went down to prepare it for sale. We were once again staying with John and Deb Darragh. We appointed a Real Estate Agent. It was a tough time to sell, and we were disappointed with the agent. Eventually people who we knew contacted us and we were able to negotiate a deal with them. Unfortunately, we were contracted with the Agent and still required to pay their fees. The offer was agreed subject to inspection.

I had some concerns with my left leg and I and was not happy with the vascular surgeon I had visited on the Gold Coast. Our good friend Robin Larkman researches her medical advisers very thoroughly and had treatment for her leg veins with Professor Parsi at Bondi Junction.

I managed to get an appointment with Professor Parsi in Sydney with the intent of having varicose vein treatment. Deborah came with me to see him. I explained the issues with my left leg, and he advised that the treatment would assist the blood flow but would not resolve the other problems I was having, particularly the sciatica. He asked me to remove my shirt and he said to Deborah "Would you say he has a moon face" to which she replied "Yes". "Do you think he has a buffalo hump" and she replied "Yes" again. "And would you say he was fat in the lower abdomen", "Yes". "And he has striata on his lower abdomen".

Professor then said "I think you may have Cushing's disease. And you should get scans of L4 and L5". I had never heard of the disease. Deborah had heard of it in dogs but wasn't saying anything. I believe that both Robin and the professor saved my life.

As I left the surgery, my GP Neena Singh rang me to see how I was going. She was very concerned for me. I told her Dr Parsi thought I might have Cushing's Disease and she replied "It won't be Cushing's Disease. That's very rare. I've never had a patient with it."

When we arrived back at John and Deb's that afternoon, I was straight on the internet to see what Cushing's Disease was all about. A few hours later and I was sure I had it. What's more it could be cured by some brain surgery – I was euphoric that I had found the cause of my illness and that it could be cured. A little brain surgery was nothing if it could improve my health – bring it on...

Despite Neena's scepticism, she arranged for a test to be done – she is very thorough and would always follow through on such an issue. The next week I was in Melbourne for an NDY Directors' and Managers' meeting when I received a call from Neena who told me in an incredulous voice "The test is positive."

Once again, Robin Larkman was able to recommend her Endocrinologist and I was able to get an appointment with

Chapter 12 – Gold Coast 2009 to 2013

Professor Bruce Robinson at Royal North Shore. On entry to his surgery, he said "I can see be the look of you that you have Cushing's Syndrome and since you haven't been on any steroids, it is almost certainly Cushing's Disease".

To explain this further, Cushing's Disease is one of three conditions which are termed "Cushing's Syndrome". Cushing's Disease is caused by a tumour on the pituitary gland and is a rare disease. Ectopic Cushing's is caused by a tumour somewhere in the torso, perhaps in the lungs, adrenal glands or pancreas. It is even more rare. The third type is Exogenous Cushing's which sometimes occurs in people taking artificial cortisone such as Prednisone. It has become the most common form of Cushing's Syndrome.

There is still a need to go through quite elaborate testing to positively identify the source of the problem. I was aware that Cushing's can cause psychosis, and as the testing proceeded, I felt this was happening to me. I started a diary to record what was happening to me. Whilst the diary started as a lucid document, I began to have problems keeping up the recording of what was happening. In the end, my writing was indecipherable, being more like Egyptian Hieroglyphics than English. I couldn't read it.

All the tests indicated a pituitary tumour, and I was sent for MRI and PET scans. When I visited Bruce Robinson for the results, he said "This is my worst nightmare. The tumour is not showing up on the scans". He explained that the tumour was probably no bigger than a grain of rice and was probably too small to show up on the scans.

Without being able to locate the tumour, the surgery to remove it could not be done. I had been feeling euphoric at the prospect of surgery being able to cure my disease. That instantly turned to despair. Probably the highs and lows were exaggerated by my developing psychosis.

St Patrick's Day, 17th March 2013, and Deborah and I visited the Sydney Fish Markets, a favourite haunt of ours. We went to Peter's for lunch, and I lined up to place our order. The waitress asked me what I wished to order. I could not speak – I was trying to answer but the words would not come out. Deborah had kept me in her line of sight and come over to speak to the waitress. We then sat down, my speech problem passed, and our meal arrived. The inability to speak recurred several times that day. We were back at John and Deb's that evening and made the decision to call an ambulance. We thought I might have had a stroke.

Off to the Royal North Shore where they put me through intensive testing and admitted me to the Neurological Ward. The diagnosis turned out to be that I was psychotic, and the speech problem was caused by the psychosis and cleared up in the next few days but not so the psychosis. When I was admitted into hospital, I was in a shared ward, and I was able to go for a walk around the floor. From the floor I noticed I could see my old office, the SBS studios and the ABC Film studio at Gore Hill, two old projects of mine. I decided this was some sought of omen.

Some people with mental problems hear voices. I had a full colour video which was based on The da Vinci Code written

Chapter 12 – Gold Coast 2009 to 2013

by Dan Brown and starring Tom Hanks. The hero was being pursued by an Asian crime gang. It went on each time I slept for several days. In one of my hallucinations, Tom had been injured and ended up in hospital with the crime gang closing in. I wandered around the floor trying to find a way out. An escape in my PJ's would have been interesting!

My psychosis got worse, and I was behaving very badly and confined to bed. My physical condition which was poor prior to the testing for Cushing's got decidedly worse during the testing. Psychiatrists attended to me and tried a range of drugs which did not work. My physical condition continued to deteriorate.

I remember some of the things I did at this time with a mixture of amusement and embarrassment. Certainly, I would not recommend removing your own catheter. I also would not recommend climbing out of a hospital bed when the rails are up. I had several falls attempting to do this, resulting in several stiches in toes, and a wound on the top of my foot which became infected by golden staph.

I was visited by our solicitor Dennis Staunton who is also a friend. He was handling the sale of our house. He decided I was not mentally competent to sign the transfer documents. My throwing a bottle of water at him may have assisted him in coming to that conclusion. What I never revealed was the story behind this. Due to the pain medication I was taking, I was suffering form constipation. On one occasion I asked for a suppository as Movicol was not working for me. One of the male nurses complained about it but complied. It did the trick and then there was the cleaning up to do. At that stage I could only stand using a wheely walker, and the nurse needed to clean up. He did this by pacing a towel between my leg and ripping it backward and forward several times. I was already very sore and this was excruciating. It was the only instance of cruelty I have ever suffered in a hospital. On the contrary, I am very grateful for the care hospital staff have shown to me over the years.

Dennis happened to look a bit like the nurse and that was enough for my water bottle tantrum.

At the same time, the psychiatrists decided they would like to try Electroconvulsive Technology (ECT) to resolve my psychosis. Deborah was not aware we had given each other power of attorney and so I was taken to a tribunal which declared me insane. That would not have surprised many of my friends.

The ECT worked after only a few sessions, and I quickly regained my sanity. Physically I was extremely ill. I had been psychotic for 5 weeks and would spend another 4 weeks recovering physically to the extent that I could leave hospital.

Deborah had continued to stay with John and Deb and visited me daily. Her sisters spent time in Sydney supporting her, as did my daughter, Belinda. What a harrowing time it was for her! And how lucky am I to have such a supportive wife.

The final problem for the hospital to consider was the foot injury. I was given a skin graft a couple of days prior to my intended discharge. On the day of discharge the specialist looked at my foot only to find the graft missing. One of the

Chapter 12 – Gold Coast 2009 to 2013

nurses had sent me into the shower without protecting the injury and it had washed off. I was able to be discharged from hospital and have this treated by a wounds nurse on the Gold Coast. It took many months to heal.

Deborah and I spent a few days in a rental apartment in Manly. I was unable to walk any more than a few steps and Deborah was pushing me round in a wheelchair when we went out. We headed back to the Gold Coast with me being wheeled on and off the flight.

On return to the Gold Coast, I again had internal bleeding and spent a couple of days in the old Alamanda Hospital (now Southport Private Hospital). Since I had spent some time in the hospital, I was able to attend the rehab as an outpatient. This was in early June 2013 and my 60th Birthday was on 15th July, and we had booked the Southport Yacht Club. I can remember our first night out was Rotary changeover at the end June. I was unable to stand up from the chair I was seated in. But things were progressing at rehab and Deborah is a hard taskmaster.

The aim was to walk with a cane only by my birthday. Rehab had various exercises including a set of stairs. Good foot (right) first up the stairs, weak foot (left or BILL) first down the stairs. Stepping up a kerb was quite daunting at first, and I started by finding a pole to help me. Eventually I was OK stepping straight up or down on the kerb. On my birthday I took a cane to get there but did not use it beyond that.

Chapter 13. Gold Coast 2013 to 2023

I recommenced work on a 3-day basis having been off work with my illness for 6 months. I worked mainly from home, visiting various offices as needed. I undertook a major review of our Design Guides and Technical memos, assisted in several legal cases which were current at the time. I also undertook a review of our documentation procedures and visited all offices to assess what was happening and provide training in how to thoroughly review an design.

During this time, I commenced exercising at a specialised gym which had equipment and supervision appropriate for my spinal injuries. I then went to a personal trainer where I received one on one attention. By and large I was in reasonable shape given my health situation. I returned to golf and played twice a week.

Meanwhile, Deborah became very involved with the VIEW club and has served for several years as president. VIEW clubs are women only and are set up by the Smith family to raise funds to assist children whose families cannot meet the full cost of education. Her club currently supports 20 kids. Deborah is dyslexic and was never assisted in overcoming that in her younger years. She also had a fear of public speaking which could not be avoided in her role as president. And she quickly became a very confident and competent speaker.

Chapter 13 – Gold Coast 2013 to 2023

No account of this part of my life would be complete without Red. In 2014, Deborah thought that it would be good for me to have a pet. I was recovering from the effects of Cushing's, and I agreed. Deborah's family grew up with daschunds and so we contacted Daschund Rescue. He is a "tweener", somewhere between a miniature and a full size dog.

He has been an absolute blessing. His name was Alfred, but we thought that didn't suit. We shortened it to Red which fits very well – he is Red in colour. A feature of my day is a walk down Tedder Ave with Red, and we stop for a coffee. In recent years I was in a mobile device which is a foot propelled tricycle designed for people with mobility problems.

Main Beach is very much a retirement suburb of the Gold Coast. A lot of high-rise apartments, with Tedder Ave being our commercial area. A lot of small shops, restaurants, and cafes. People are very friendly, and I find myself chatting to people throughout our morning stroll. I was identified by Red and by my bright yellow tricycle. In the past couple of months, I have been on a power scooter and my missing left leg attracts a bit of attention.

Believe it or not, Red writes poetry and has a book of poems. To explain how this works, this is the "Message from the author" Red provided:

I decided to write some poems about my life and experiences. I have included stories involving my humans (Dee Dee and Poppa) and other humans in my life.

As you can imagine, it is very difficult for me to write or type anything – paws are bloody useless in that way.

I thought of asking Dee Dee to write type them, but she is a dyslexic agnostic insomniac who lies awake all night wondering if there is a dog.

I tell Poppa what to write. He's not very bright but he is able to get the job done with liberal use of spellcheck.

If I have offended anyone, that's tough luck – suck it up.

This one is based on the day Dee Dee and Poppa picked up Red

Red the Rescue

I was born on a Toowoomba Farm
And sold to a young guy
Who decided he didn't want me
I'm cute and wonder why

Back to the farm I was taken
And a daschund rescue became
Dee Dee and Pop wanted a wiener
And happily staked their claim

They came to Toowoomba to get me
And had a cake and some tea
I growled at first at Poppa
But I really liked Dee Dee.

Chapter 13 – Gold Coast 2013 to 2023

And then it was time to leave
The car door opened, I jumped on the seat
Cars are my favourite things
I think they are really neat.

We drove all the way to Main Beach
And I am a lucky guy
From an unwanted puppy rescue
I moved to a house in the sky.

One of the poems related to an infamous incident at our local coffee shop. It involved our very good friend Mick. Mick and his partner Kerri stay in our unit and baby sit Red when Deborah and I are off on one of our frequent holidays.

The Fable of the Table

Mick walked to Crema and had a dilemma,
How to stop me harassing a hound,
The leg of the table seemed to be able
To restrain me – a theory unsound.

Mick went for his cup as I sighted a pup
A fluffy walking down Tedder
I dragged the table which wasn't able
To stop me – I went off to get her.

People stopped their chatter at the mighty clatter
The table toppled and was dragged down the road
Pandemonium resulted as the white fluffy bolted
Chased by me and my table load.

That's the score, now its Tedder folk law
They all seem to know the fable
The story's more bold each time it is told
And I earned the Red Terror label.

During latter years, I have had increasingly suffered mobility problems. These started with the golf ball injury in 2008, sciatica in both legs starting in 2008, followed by the DVT in 2011, then an achilles rupture in 2012. The achilles rupture prevented me from walking quickly. Sciatica was painful, but I learned various exercises which helped, and I also recovered if I stopped for a while. Following my hospitalisation in 2013, I couldn't walk. Following rehab, I was able to walk again - say 3 km with Red in the mornings and I could play golf albeit in a cart. Throughout the whole period I continued gym workouts. Nonetheless, my muscles continued to atrophy, and this seemed to accelerate around 2018 to 2022. My bone density actually improved in this time – I was taking Prolia injections and was on a high protein diet as well as the gym work.

In January 2017 Deborah and I flew to Africa for a holiday which included Victoria falls. The tour ended in Capetown, where we stayed for a couple of days before catching the Queen Mary for a cruise to Fremantle. We went to Geraldton to stay with Deborah's sister Margaret and her husband Scott. During the stay I managed to fall down their stairs which were tiles with a steel edge. I managed to put a large gash in my arm and crush a vertebra in my back. I went to Geraldton Hospital by ambulance.

Chapter 13 – Gold Coast 2013 to 2023

It took a few days to repair my arm and X-rays were taken of my back. Somehow the doctors thought the fracture was an old one and did nothing about it and did not advise me. After several months of pain, I attended a specialist on the Gold Coast who found the fracture. By then the injury was healed and there was no problem. About this time the sciatic pain I had suffered for ten years was relieved and has not since return. Could it be that the latest injury moved things around and taken the pressure off the nerves?

I advised the Geraldton Hospital of the issue. They checked it out and advised that they were in error and apologised for the incident.

One of the muscle loss areas was on the soles of my feet on the padding which protects the leg bone. This was an extremely painful condition and put me at risk of stress fractures. It caused me to give up golf. In 2021, I purchased an Alinker which is a three wheeled tricycle – two at the front and on small wheel at the rear. There are no pedals, you must use your feet to propel it. Your sit quite upright on the seat, which is far better psychologically than being in a scooter or a wheelchair. It actually requires more physical effort than walking, so contributed to aerobic fitness.

The deterioration in my muscles and the pain I was suffering prompted a reconsideration of the treatment for my Cushing's disease and Professor Robinson believed I should have my adrenal glands removed. This is the most radical of the treatments for treating Cushing's but probably appropriate in my case. So I was programmed for the operation.

Not long after I got the Alinker, I saw a newsclip on Channel 7 on a group called Now I Can Run. This featured a number of wheelchair bound kids and young people who were racing a foot propelled tricycle a little like the Alinker. However, I would describe my device as a Camry compared to their Ferraris. Known generally as a RaceRunner, the devices are raced competitively by handicapped people. They are under consideration for the Paralympics.

The kids have such conditions as Spina Bifida, Cerebral Palsy and Muscular Dystrophy. Whilst they have limited ability to walk, they are able to propel a RaceRunner as soon as they hop on one. The delight they have in riding and racing their trike is wonderful to see and very contagious. They get a form of physical exercise unequalled by anything else they can do. The mental stimulation they receive is very obvious.

I contacted their CEO Amy Tobin who is wheelchair bound and a very accomplished RaceRunner. She and her carer Drew are dedicated to promoting RaceRunning and involving young handicapped kids in the sport. At my suggestion the Rotary Club had Amy and Drew along as guest speakers. We also made a donation which enabled a young boy to own a RaceRunner.

I discussed an idea with Deborah that we should hold an Art Sale on the top floor of our apartment, and suggested

Chapter 13 – Gold Coast 2013 to 2023

it as a Rotary Club Project, which was agreed to. The area is quite large and set up for entertaining. We invited Donald Waters to display his artwork which he was most willing to do. He also donated a beautiful artwork which we had an online auction for. Donald is very community minded and supports a lot of charities and has been awarded an Order of Australia Medal. One of his annual activities is to visit the streets in his area dressed up as Santa conveyed by the local Bush Fire Brigade. Donald has a close resemblance to St Nick, complete with full snowy white beard. I am told some of the donations are in liquid form and used to lubricate the participants over the Christmas period.

As the date for the Art Sale approached, things became confused as the date for my adrenal gland operation started shifting around. It was originally programmed for Tuesday 1st March 2022 but delayed when one of the medical team had COVID and was reprogrammed to Friday 18th March with the Art Show locked in on Sunday 20th March, when I would be in hospital. As happens in my wife's family, the SOS call went out to the Hockey girls, and they responded. Judith arrived all the way from Perth. Our good friend Robin also flew in from Sydney. And, of course the Rotary Club was available.

At the last minute, my operation was again cancelled. This time there were some problems with the operating theatres. The operation actually went ahead on the Tuesday after the Art Show. So, I could attend, which was wonderful. We had the show open all afternoon and people came and went as they pleased. Besides the original art works, there were some reproductions, and beach towels and cushion covers produced from Donald's paintings. Former NDY CEO and very good friend Ian Hopkins provided his very fine Tellurian wines for tasting.

One of the attendees had recently bought a 4 storey Penthouse in Surfers Paradise and commissioned Donald for a very large painting to suit a 2 storey high wall. I was very pleased to see him do well from the day, particularly since he had been so generous.

The Rotary Club was able to donate $4,500 to Now I Can Run which was used to purchase a RaceRunner for Caleb, a young man with cerebral palsy who had recently taken up the sport. He had already been successful, winning local, state, national and Oceania events. Some Rotarians visited the Now I Can Run training sessions at Griffith University to officially hand over to RaceRunner, and to see the kids in action. Caleb was taken to the event by his grandmother, and both thanked us for the trike. Grandma explained that RaceRunning had totally changed Caleb's view on life and attitude.

And then there was Sandra, a tiny 5-year-old girl who was on her own (very small) RaceRunner and was not going to get off. She could propel herself very well and obviously greatly enjoyed doing so. Her propulsion skills did exceed her navigation skills and Mum was required to help.

I found the Alinker very exhausting over long distances and investigated an alternative. I ended up buying a motorised scooter which folds up into the equivalent of an in-cabin

Chapter 13 – Gold Coast 2013 to 2023

bag. I use it for travel and for long distance trips near home. As I was having trouble walking up stairs, I purchased a stair climber to get me to the upper floor of our apartment.

Given this deterioration, my endocrinologist thought I needed to have my adrenal glands removed, which would stop me producing cortisol, therefore cure my Cushing's disease. I would then have Addison's disease, the treatment for which is taking artificial cortisone.

I finally underwent my laparoscopic bilateral adrenalectomy three days after the Art Show. I woke up in intensive care to discover only my left adrenal gland had been removed. Something had gone astray with the operation, and it had taken far too long, and I was under stress.

As this was happening, I started looking at the Australian Pituitary Foundation (APF) which is a support and advocacy group for sufferers of Pituitary diseases. I was impressed with the information available and thought I should join which I did in late 2021. I also volunteered to be on the Fundraising and Communications Sub Committee.

In late 2022, my Rotary Club generously donated use of our Chapel (which we hire out for weddings, etc) for an awareness session on pituitary diseases. The MD of the APF, spoke generally on the topic and specifically on her daughter Ruby who was born with a non-functional pituitary and was a very ill baby until the condition was diagnosed. She requires daily cortisone tablets and injections of growth hormone. After lobbying by the APF the government allowed weekly growth injections and funds these. Ruby is a very cute little girl and generally is very well and active. Great care must be taken when she catches any virus as her medication may not be effective.

I spoke on the trials and tribulations of a Cushing's sufferer and a friend and fellow Cushy Maree Brady spoke on her experiences. Like myself Maree suffered psychosis and was in an institution when her psychiatrist diagnosed her with Cushing's disease. She was able to have her tumour removed and after a lengthy recovery managed to get back to a healthy life.

We were also fortunate to have Dr Wayne Ng, neurologist speak on the treatment for pituitary patients.

Rotary District Governor Karen Thomas has a medical background and was present. She asked me to make a similar presentation to the Rotary District conference in Yamba in May 2023.

I was appointed to the APF board in November 2022

Finding a time when the two surgeons, the anaesthetist and I were all free from COVID and were available proved very difficult and there was a delay of three months until the surgery could be completed. Give the previous experience, the anaesthetist took additional precautions. The second operation went better than the first but was still difficult. Another two days in intensive care.

Within a couple of days, I felt decidedly better than I could ever remember. My vision seemed much brighter. I think

Chapter 13 – Gold Coast 2013 to 2023

this was due to getting of ketoconazole which is quite a dirty drug. My finger and toenails had been splitting badly and were now improving. The skin on my arms and legs improved rapidly. I enjoyed this for a couple of months.

Between the two surgeries, Deborah and I enjoyed a Tasmanian cruise. It was at a time when COVID was rampant, but we were fortunate that the cruise went ahead and there were no health issues. There was a change to our intended itinerary and the cruise was based on hiking and hill/mountain climbing and I could not participate in many of the activities. However, we enjoyed ourselves on the cruise and during our extended time in Hobart.

I then suffered the infection of the toes and vascular calcification resulting in the amputation of my left leg as described in chapter 1. I was fortunate to have had the adrenalectomy as my skin condition when I had Cushing's would have been too poor to have allowed the amputation to be successfully done – the "stump" wound would not have healed.

Chapter 14. Rantings of an Old Man

How I Have Changed.
It would be difficult to go through what I have without being affected by my experiences. I will leave out the physical illnesses and injuries which are simply something which I must cope with.

The real differences are the changes in attitude and how that plays out. Whilst I of course knew that our time on this planet is limited, I think I didn't emotionally accept that until I went through my first life threatening experience. I think that increased my determination to enjoy life, contribute to the communities I was am part of and be more relaxed.

I have from 2011 when I ruptured my achilles had increasing mobility problems and by 2020 had succumbed to mobility devices to assist me. This took a turn for the worse when I had to have my left leg amputated.

Overall, people are very kind and considerate and able to lend a hand when I have a problem. Sometimes my scooter gets jammed on a culvert linking a footpath to a street crossing and other times Red's lead gets tangled in the wheels. People are willing to help. Last Christmas Day I was out with Red early in the morning when the scooter

Chapter 14 – Rantings of an Old Man

stopped, and I could not get it going. I had forgotten to bring my mobile phone and was stranded. A lady was kind enough to lend me her phone so I could ring Deborah and have her rescue me.

There are some annoyances, which are always due to lack of thought not malice. The fact that my head is at a low height often means that I am not seen. I need to be careful in crowds as people are likely to run into me. Many shops and reception desks have high counters and even if my head is visible above counter level, the person behind the counter does not pick that up because their mind is attuned to the customer at a higher level. It reminds me of my childhood when I couldn't be seen above the lolly counter.

Occasionally I will get the circumstance where I ask a question of someone, and they respond to my wife. I think people of my generation were brought up thinking that a person in a wheelchair is lacking in intelligence. I think they may also feel awkward in dealing with handicapped people. Whilst I am sure attitudes have changed, old habits are hard to break. I have had to learn to be tolerant and understanding.

The few months after my leg amputation have tested my patience. I have always been inclined to get things done as soon as possible and be frustrated when I can't. Now my disability means some things take a lot longer and it is a battle to do get used to this new reality. My mobility problems stop me from doing a lot a things I would like to be doing, and the need to keep my legs raised also confines me to a chair. I find myself watching a lot more TV than I would like. I undertook the writing of this book which would never have happened without my incapacitation.

I am very fortunate that a prosthetic will remove many of the issues outlined above. And experiencing these issues provides me with a valuable insight into how wheelchair bound people feel.

I have been through a major mental breakdown and many physical problems and a few life-threatening experiences. These have great value in proving me with empathy for those who are doing it tough. My father was a major influence on me in this area, but my depth of empathy has increased significantly due to my own experiences.

Treatment of disabled people.
I think Australia is a world leader in our treatment of disabled people and disabled people are making an outstanding contribution to our community. Our disabled athletes are very prominent in the Paralympics, the Invictus games, tennis, and other handicapped sports.

The support available from the Government through the National Disability Insurance Scheme (NDIS) has done a great deal in enriching the lives of disabled people, their carers and their families.

I find it disturbing that NDIS is not available to person 65 and over. This was done to reduce the cost of the system and the burden that would have on the taxpayer. It is a clear case of age discrimination and needs to be re-examined.

Chapter 14 – Rantings of an Old Man

I think perhaps NDIS should be means tested on a basis consistent with pensions. Those of us who are wealthy enough to be self-funded retirees would not be eligible. At the moment a person who is say 66 and becomes disabled has no access to the scheme and may not have the financial capacity to pay for equipment and services available under NDIS and not under My Aged Care.

People who inspire.
I can't put an exact timeline on my disability as a I had increasing mobility problems over recent years, with the amputation being an unwelcome shock in the last few months. As this has been occurring, I have looked for people who have overcome their disabilities and lived a positive and productive life.

Wheelchair tennis player Dylan Alcott springs to mind as a great athlete with a wonderful personality and sporting attitude who was Australian of the year in 2022. At birth, he had a tumour wrapped around his spinal cord, which he had cut out at just a couple of days old, leaving him with his disability. Not only was he the dominant wheelchair tennis player of his time, he also won paralympic gold in wheelchair basketball. His attitude is that he is glad to have his handicap as it has made him into what he is today.

I recently spoke at a conference where two inspirational disabled people spoke. First up was Dr Dinesh Palipana who is a quadriplegic doctor. His injuries occurred early in his university medical studies, and he competed the majority of his course and subsequent internship despite of the challenges he faced. He also had to fight the medical bureaucracy some elements of which sought to exclude him based on his handicap.

The second handicapped speaker was Curtis McGrath. Curtis lost both his legs due to a land mine in Afghanistan where he served with the Australian Army. Curtis was a trained medic and as he was being carried to a location to rendezvous with a helicopter, he instructed his mates on how to save his life. Prior to being place in the helicopter, he announced that he would be competing in the Paralympics. He won gold in canoeing events In Rio De Janeiro and Tokyo. I was still awaiting my prosthetic at the time and had come some way in learning to cope with life with one leg amputated. He had to deal with dual amputations which he did with great courage and determination. I was programmed to speak a little later and had a chat with him and looked and his prostheses.

The other person I admire is Sophie Delezio who with her friend Mollie was horribly burnt when a car crashed into their kindergarten and exploded into flames. They were only 3 years old at the time. Sophie had burns to 90% of her body and lost a leg. It was a miracle she lived, and the press followed her story closely. I was supportive of the fundraising efforts made which went for the hospital where she was a patient. From that very early age, Sophie came across as very confident and resilient and this applies to the present day. Her father Ron set up the Day of Difference Foundation which assists children with injuries and their families.

Sophie, Curtis, and Dinesh believe their handicaps are essential ingredients in them becoming the people they

Chapter 14 – Rantings of an Old Man

are today. I understand that and feel that my various problems have contributed to the person I now am.

Our Health System

I am very grateful for the treatment I have been given by the medical staff who have looked after me. There are major stresses on the system as it tries to cope with an aging population. And the more successful they are at prolonging lives, the greater the workload becomes. And the ethnic mix of the staff in the system demonstrates clearly how much immigrants to this county are contributing.

Rare Diseases.

The area where I have concerns about our system is in the diagnosis of rare diseases and in particular the early diagnosis of these diseases. Not that I think the performance in Australia is any worse than other nations. I do not have the qualifications the speak with authority generally but have looked closely at the length of time to diagnose Cushing's disease and I would think similar issues arise with other rare conditions.

There are over 7,000 known rare diseases and more are being identified each year. With that in mind, I have great sympathy for the doctors who have no chance of being knowledgeable on each of these conditions. When I started displaying symptoms of Cushing's none of the health professionals I visited had treated a Cushing's patient. I think even one of them had suspected a hormonal problem, I would have been referred to an Endocrinologist and I would almost certainly have been correctly diagnosed. I struck it lucky when a vascular surgeon who had a penchant for diagnosis made a preliminary diagnosis and I was on my way to treating the underlying problem. My case is by no means unusual. Many sufferers have similar time to diagnose, and it is now accepted that people are dying from Cushing's without being diagnosed – I was fortunate not to be one of them.

The system basically works like this:

A GP directly looks after the readily identifiable and treatable problems. A more complex problem is referred to a specialist. Should there be several complex problems, the patient is referred to several different specialists. Specialists tend to look in their area of expertise and treat the problem in isolation. We do have physicians who are skilled in diagnosing complex conditions. I went to a physician for many years, and he was unable to diagnose the problem. I think we are dealing with too many complex conditions for any one person to keep up with all the conditions we are talking about.

In the case of complex conditions, I don't believe this approach is working (whilst freely admitting I have no medical training).

I have been fortunate enough to have private health insurance and have been able to afford the considerable costs involved in seeing the best of specialists. I am concerned that a person without health cover and limited income would not be so lucky and their chance of survival would be substantially reduced.

Chapter 15. The Future

For me it is important to consider the future and make plans which consider the issues with my health

My right leg is of considerable concern – as Venu Bhamidi, the Vascular Surgeon who performed the amputation of "Bill" so directly and eloquently put it "The veins in your right leg are crap." I must be extremely careful not to injure my right foot (the only one I have left to injure), because healing of any injury would be very problematic. There is a very real possibility that I could lose my right leg in the future. I am not going to plan around that but will change my plans if it occurs to address the altered reality.

I have been under the treatment of Dr John Meulet for my heart issues for many years and have been regularly tested and the results have been consistently favourable. Given that the veins in my legs are so poor, the obvious issue was the condition of the veins in my heart. Testing for this type of problem would normally involve a stress test which is done on a treadmill. Since I have a leg missing this is not feasible for me.

I did my own little test using a piece of gym equipment similar to a grinding wheel on a yacht. I use this for 20 minutes as part of my regular physio session. My heart rate after the test was only slightly elevated above resting. Not very scientific but it gave me some optimism while I waited for more elaborate testing to be done. Subsequently I have done a CT scan which picks up the calcium build up around the heart. It indicates the arteries have been restricted by about 25 %. As this test is not very accurate, I then did an angiogram whereby a probe is injected into the wrist and manoeuvred into the blood vessels around the heart. Fortunately, this all looks quite good and my heart should not be a problem for the foreseeable future.

The strange thing for me is that my cholesterol has been low for all my life other than in 2008 when it was a little high due to undiagnosed Cushing's. Since then, I have been on medication which has kept the level very low. I have queried several times whether I should discontinue the medication. Dr John's response has been that he wants to keep the level low given my history of clotting and atrial fibrillation. Even though my latest cholesterol level was 3.5, my medication has been doubled. Evidently having a low level may help dissolve some of the plaque.

Given the vagaries of the above, it is time to make hay while the sun shines. I look forward to the removal of the restrictions imposed on me due to my confinement to a wheelchair or mobility scooter. Simple things like being able to reach goods on a high shelf or at the rear of a cupboard. Being able to step over a small step and access our decks to have breakfast overlooking the beach and the Broadwater. Do a bit of gardening, get to the BBQ, or use our spa tub. I will remain in our apartment as long as is practical.

Chapter 15 – The Future

As I write this final chapter, I have just had my prosthesis fitted for the first time and I will be going back to the rehab Hospital to see that all is well and to train me in how to walk in it. I did some walking this morning and it all went very well. This will also give me the ability to drive my car alone, and if necessary, load a mobility device in and out. All these things take a considerable load off Deborah. Caring for me has taken up a lot or her time and has caused her considerable back pain.

Golf is certainly on the agenda. I think it will require considerable rehabilitation and the right type of prosthetic. If I can achieve my golfing ambitions, I think I will be able to swim both in the local swimming pool and in the surf. I will walk with Red (our daschund) for morning coffee and along the beach. These activities have been denied to me in recent years due to the problems with my legs, and my left leg. They were very much taken for granted – it is only when I have been denied them that I realise how important they are.

I will return to playing bridge which is an activity which is not reliant on my mobility (other than getting there) and is certainly good for my mental condition.

We have in the past had many holidays. Of latter years, as we have become less physically active, these have tended to be cruises. We currently have bookings for cruises from Hawaii to Brisbane, from Auckland to Sydney and from Cairns to Cairns.

Maintaining contact with family and friends is important. A busy social life is also ensured – Deborah is very much the organiser in this area. Children and grandchildren are an important part.

My community work is very much centred around Rotary, and I intend to remain an active member of the club. I currently am working on the local production of RaceRunners, a tricycle which handicapped children get to propel by foot. They are extremely expensive, and I am convinced we can provide them at a much lower price via a not-for-profit organisation. I am working with Griffith University who are designing the device. We also need to set up a business entity to handle the manufacture, assembly, marketing, and accounting of the Race Runners. Besides being a very worthwhile thing to do, it is a challenge for me and a distraction from health concerns which may occur.

Acknowledgements

Firstly I thank Professor Kurosh Parsi who diagnosed my Cushing's disease within 5 mins pf seeing me, ending many years of suffering from an undiagnosed illness. He saved my life. I also thank endocrinologist Professor Bruce Robinson AM has treated me through 10 years of coping with my illness.

My GP Neena Singh who told me "It won't be Cushing's. That's very rare". Then, being the professional she is, she arranged for me to have a test which to her surprise came out positive. And to all the doctors, nursing staff, physios and other hospital staff who have looked after me. We call Australia the lucky country and we are very lucky to have our health system.

To all my colleagues, partners and friends at NDY, thank you for providing me with so many challenges and opportunities. These have provided me with a very rewarding career which has been fundamental to coping with the illness I have suffered. I also thank the many fellow professional I have worked with over many years.

For the Rotary colleagues I have served with for over 40 years of membership in four different clubs, it has been a privilege to work with you.

Our friends and family have been a great support not only to me but also to Deborah.

Most of all I thank Deborah for being my carer which has taken its toll at various times both physically and mentally.

www.ingramcontent.com/pod-product-compliance
Lightning Source LLC
Chambersburg PA
CBHW032054090426
42744CB00005B/209